THE BEGINNER'S GUIDE TO
STRENGTH TRAINING
— FOR —
WOMEN OVER 50

- ✓ **Flexible** 30 Minute Workouts
- ✓ **Improve Your** Mobility
- ✓ **Crush Menopausal Weight Gain**
- ✓ **Unlock a More** Vibrant **You**

Includes Nutrition and Yoga to
Complement Your Journey

SAGE LIFESTYLE PRESS

Disclaimer and Waiver:

The information presented in this book is intended for educational purposes only and is not intended to diagnose, treat, cure, or prevent any disease. The contents of this book are based on the author's personal research, experiences, and opinions. Before beginning any new exercise, nutrition, or health program, consult your physician or other qualified health professional to ensure it is appropriate for your individual circumstances, especially if you have pre-existing medical conditions or are taking medications.

The author and publisher of this book are not responsible for any injuries or health conditions that may result from following the recommendations, advice, or exercises described herein. Use of the information in this book is at your own risk. Always listen to your body and discontinue any exercise that causes pain or discomfort.

Waiver

By participating in any exercise program or activity described in this book, you acknowledge and agree to the following:

1. You have consulted with your physician or other qualified health professional regarding your ability to engage in physical exercise without risking harm to your health.

2. You understand that physical exercise involves inherent risks, including but not limited to the risk of injury, heart attack, stroke, or other serious conditions.

3. You voluntarily assume all risks associated with physical exercise and fully accept responsibility for any injury, harm, or loss that may result.

4. You release and discharge the author, publisher, and any associated parties from any and all claims or causes of action, known or unknown, arising from the use of the information, advice, or exercises contained in this book.

By using this book, you agree to the terms of this waiver and disclaimer. If you do not agree, please refrain from using the information and exercises provided in this book.

Acknowledgment

The world is a better place thanks to individuals who strive to develop and lead others to overcome obstacles. Those who generously sharing their knowledge and time to mentor and educate are even more valuable. I want to express my gratitude to Joanne Lee Cornish, a woman who embodies these qualities.

Joanne is not just a personal coach but a source of inspiration and a champion of healthy body composition. Her coaching and guidance, particularly in her masterclasses, have been instrumental in transforming my body. Her focus on midlife, supportive approach, and unwavering encouragement set her apart.

I highly recommend her book "When Calories & Cardio Don't Cut It: Know What Influences Your Body Weight and Shape so That You Can Live Lean for a Lifetime" at https://www.amazon.com/dp/B07L5Z6VRP.

You can also connect with her at https://linktr.ee/Theshrinkshop and on IG @joanneleecornish.

Other acknowledgments:

Cover design by The Creative Pulse,
https://99designs.com/profiles/thecreativepulse,
with cover images from istockphoto.com (left to right)
by kali9, gzorgz, luengo, Tinpixels, digitalskillet, and Milan Markovic.

Illustrations created by dienart92

Table of Contents

Introduction **6**

Chapter 1: Getting Started with Strength Training..................**8**

   1.1 Why Strength Training Is So Important 9

   1.2 Overcoming the Myth: "I'm Too Old to Start Strength Training" 9

   1.3 Understanding Your Body's Changes 12

   1.4 Setting Up Your Home Gym with Minimum Equipment.................14

   1.5 Tailoring Your Space for Safe Training 15

   1.6 The First Step: Fitness Assessment 16

Chapter 2: The Beginner Strength Training Routine...................**24**

Chapter 3: Exercise Modifications..................................**47**

   3.1 Low-impact Strength Training: Safe for Arthritis 47

   3.2 Exercises to Enhance Bone Density Post Menopause....................49

   3.3 Adapting Workouts for Reduced Mobility 49

   3.4 Strength Training with Osteoporosis: A Detailed Guide 51

   3.5 Building Core Strength for Better Balance and Stability 52

   3.6 Customizing Workouts: When and How to Modify Exercises...........55

Chapter 4: Nutrition, Recovery, and Weight Loss.....................**57**

   4.1 Nutrition Essentials: Eating for Muscle Recovery....................57

   4.2 The Role of Hydration in Effective Strength Training 60

   4.3 Supplements: What Helps and What Doesn't? 61

   4.4 Understanding and Managing Post-workout Soreness 63

   4.5 Sleep's Role in Muscle Recovery 65

   4.6 Active Recovery Techniques..66

   4.7 Menopausal Weight Gain and Nutritional Needs 70

Chapter 5: Next Steps—Building Your Routine 80

5.1 Designing Your Weekly Strength Training Plan.............................. 80

5.2 Integrating Strength Training with Other Types of Exercise............................81

5.3 Setting Realistic Goals and Milestones 82

5.4 When to Upscale Your Exercises.. 84

Chapter 6: Advanced Techniques and Strategies...............................86

6.1 Incorporating Resistance Bands into Your Routine........................... 86

6.2 Advanced Workout Options 87

6.3 Exploring High-intensity Low-impact Training (HILIT) 99

6.4 Progressive Overload: What It Is and How to Use It.........................100

6.5 Leveraging Technology for Enhanced Training...............................102

Chapter 7: Connecting the Mind and Body 104

7.1 Mindfulness and Meditation for Strength Trainers 104

7.2 The Psychological Benefits of Regular Exercise...............................106

7.3 Stress Reduction through Physical Activity 108

7.4 Yoga and Pilates: Complementary Practices for Strength Training 109

7.5 The Power of Positive Thinking in Fitness 112

7.6 Building Mental Resilience through Routine Exercise 113

Chapter 8: Long-term Health and Wellness...............................115

8.1 Managing Chronic Conditions with Regular Exercise 115

8.2 The Lifelong Benefits of Maintaining Muscle Mass............................ 116

8.3 Preventing Falls and Injuries through Targeted Exercises...............................117

8.4 Planning for a Healthy Future: Beyond Strength Training 119

Conclusion 122

References 124

Introduction

As women approach midlife, they often feel more and less confident. They admit they feel free from the insecurities of their youth while struggling with changes in their appearance. This change can make it hard to find a new identity that is not dependent on how others see them.

As I passed my 60th birthday, I saw many ads online promising to make me look younger and more beautiful. Society expects women to dislike their aging faces and bodies, spending lots of time and money on anti-aging products and procedures. If you see through the tricks and want to decide that feeling good and being healthy is the ultimate goal, then keep reading because strength training is the panacea. Maintaining strength and vitality regardless of age will become your new mantra, and we at Sage Lifestyle Press are here to guide you!

Five years ago, I found myself very sick very quickly. I was diagnosed with Acute Myeloid Leukemia (AML, or blood cancer). I was healthy; at 55 years old, I did weight training and aerobic walking, and I was proud of my ability to climb stairs without getting winded and carry my groceries easily. However, sometimes, life gets in the way, and I found myself on a journey that no one could have predicted.

After a long struggle with cancer, I re-entered the fitness arena. Even though I have a background in health and fitness and know that getting back to a solid exercise routine that included strength training would be beneficial, I still needed to employ all the guidance I'm sharing in this book. Now, I am back to strength training and walking as I regain my strength. The road back has been difficult, but I remember one thing from a disease that kills more people than survive it—if I weren't in such good health, my outcome would likely have been very different. This pivotal moment underscored a vital truth: strength training after 50 isn't just beneficial but a must for all women.

This book is founded on the belief that strength training goes beyond maintaining physical health—it's about reclaiming and enhancing your vitality, independence, and self-assurance. Here, you'll uncover the physical benefits, such as improved bone density and muscle maintenance, as well as significant boosts to your mental health and overall quality of life.

Many midlife women shy away from strength training due to fears of injury or the misconception that it's too late to start. This book aims to dismantle those fears by providing reliable information and practical strategies. We'll navigate these hurdles together, backed by scientific research and expert opinions, ensuring you feel safe and informed.

The Midlife Guide to Strength Training for Women is more than just a book; it's a comprehensive guide designed to accompany you on your journey into strength training. Combining practical exercises, nutritional advice, and motivational tools, this book offers a structured yet flexible approach to fitness.

What sets this guide apart is its focus on needs specific to our age group. It includes age-appropriate exercises and modifications to accommodate various health conditions and addresses the psychological impact of aging on fitness. If, like me, you are recovering from an illness, you will find the support you need to take that first step.

My passion for writing this book stems from personal experience and a heartfelt desire to assist others. Having navigated the challenges and rewards of strength training, I am eager to share this knowledge.

As we embark on this journey together, let this book be your mentor and motivator. It's always possible to start, and our path is filled with potential for rediscovery and empowerment. Let's lift not only weights, but also our spirits and aspirations.

I invite you to turn the page and join me in transforming our lives through strength training. Together, we will explore how embracing this path can lead to a healthier, more vibrant, and empowered version of ourselves.

Ready to feel your best? Let's get started.

1

Getting Started with Strength Training

Have you heard someone say, "I wish I had started earlier"? Many of us share a common sentiment regarding caring for our health and fitness. But here's a little secret that might change how you think about embarking on a new fitness regime, especially strength training: it's always possible to start. The benefits of picking up strength training could be even more significant than ever imagined. This chapter will guide you to embrace strength training, dispel myths, and set you up for success.

Experts widely recommend strength training as the most critical exercise activity in midlife. Strength training, also known as resistance training, helps maintain muscle mass, which tends to decline with age and improves bone density, balance, and metabolic health. This type of exercise can significantly enhance functional fitness, making daily activities easier and reducing the risk of falls and injuries.

Many types of exercise are helpful. However, if time is limited, prioritizing strength training can provide significant health benefits. The National Institute on Aging (NIA) also emphasizes the importance of strength training for older adults. Research supported by the NIA indicates that strength training builds muscle mass and reduces muscle mass loss, which maintains mobility and independence.

According to the American College of Sports Medicine (ACSM), regular resistance exercise reduces the risk of numerous diseases, improves quality of life, and decreases mortality rates. Their guidelines suggest that adults engage in strength training exercises involving major muscle groups at least two to three times per week.

A 2002 study by the University of Arizona found that "resistance and weight-bearing exercise had a significant and positive impact on post-menopausal women's total and regional body composition." Additionally, resistance training can reduce hot flashes in post-menopausal women.

1.1 Why Strength Training Is So Important

As we get older, it's normal to lose muscle. This starts in our 30s, with adults losing about 3% to 8% of their muscle each decade. After age 50, muscle loss speeds up to 5% to 10% per decade. For women, menopause makes this worse because the drop in estrogen causes faster muscle loss and more fat gain.

Muscle burns more calories than fat, even when you're resting. For example, a pound of muscle uses about six calories per day at rest, while a pound of fat uses only about two calories daily. This means muscle is three times more active in burning calories compared to fat, helping to boost your metabolism.

The best way to slow down this process and gain muscle after menopause is to practice strength training. Lifting weights builds muscle, increases strength, and helps with balance and agility. You can use gym machines, free weights, resistance bands, or your body weight.

Many people think they need more aerobic exercise to lose weight, but more muscle mass boosts your metabolism. Weight loss can include muscle loss without strength training, but lifting weights helps maintain muscle while losing fat.

1.2 Overcoming the Myth: "I'm Too Old to Start Strength Training"

In our society, there's a pervasive myth that once you hit a certain age, it's too late to start something new, particularly physically demanding activities like strength training. However, scientific research robustly supports the benefits of lifting weights, especially for women in midlife. Studies indicate regular strength training can enhance bone density, combat age-related muscle loss, and significantly boost your metabolic rate.

Moreover, it's been shown to improve sleep quality, mental health, and overall life satisfaction. These findings are crucial, especially considering the natural physical decline that can come with age. They underscore that introducing strength training into your routine can be a game-changer, helping to reverse or mitigate some of these declines.

Osteopenia is a condition where your bones are weaker than when you were younger but not so weak that they break easily, like osteoporosis. It's like a warning sign that your bones are losing strength, and you need to take steps to keep them healthy.

Many women worry that strength training will make them bulky, but this isn't true because women have much less testosterone than men (only ~10%). Instead, strength training helps women look more toned and trimmer.

Embracing this new or renewed chapter in your fitness life is about more than just the physical benefits. It's equally about shifting your mindset. The belief that you're "too old" to start strength training is a significant barrier. Overcoming this starts with changing how you talk about your abilities and potential. This mental shift will permeate all areas of your life. Remember, the goal here isn't to compete with what you could do at 30 but to build a stronger, more resilient body that serves you well today.

Journaling

Keeping a fitness and nutrition journal offers the following benefits:

- **Tracking Progress:** This allows you to monitor your improvements over time, such as increased strength, endurance, and flexibility. Nutrition tracking can show how your eating habits affect your workouts and overall health.

- **Motivation:** Logging your progress provides a tangible way to see progress and can encourage you to stick with your fitness and nutrition routines.

- **Accountability:** Writing down your workouts and goals helps keep you accountable to yourself.

- **Identifying Patterns:** You can determine what works best for you by looking at patterns in your exercise routines and their results. These notes can help you adjust as needed.

- **Setting Goals:** Journaling helps you set and track specific, measurable goals.

- **Reflecting on Successes and Challenges:** This practice provides you a space to reflect on what you've accomplished and any obstacles you've faced, helping you to make adjustments as needed.

- **Staying Organized:** It keeps your fitness plan organized, making it easier to follow and adjust.

- **Mental Health Benefits:** Journaling can also provide mental health benefits, such as stress reduction and a sense of accomplishment.

You don't need anything fancy here; a simple wire-bound notebook will do. Now, take a moment to jot down your fears or hesitations about starting strength training. Next to each, write a positive counterstatement. For example, if you wrote, "I might get hurt," counter it with, "I will learn the proper techniques and start with light weights to ensure I stay safe." This exercise is about planning and actively reshaping your thoughts toward strength training.

Remember, this journey isn't about willpower but building a habit. Just like ensuring you brush your teeth, you can find time for your overall health and vitality. Building an exercise habit can be challenging, but it can become an integral part of your daily routine with the right strategies. Here are some of the best ways to build and maintain an exercise habit:

1. **Schedule Workouts:** Treat exercise like any other important appointment. Schedule it in your calendar and stick to it.

2. **Choose Exercises You Enjoy**: Find fun and enjoyable exercises. This book has provided a beginner workout plan, but you can mix and match. I particularly like deadlifts. Doing something you love increases the likelihood of sticking with it. You can find deadlifts in the advanced workouts section in Chapter 5.

3. **Track Your Progress:** Monitor your progress using a journal, app, or wearable fitness tracker. Seeing improvements can boost motivation.

4. **Prepare Ahead of Time:** Lay out your workout clothes and equipment the night before. This will reduce excuses and make it easier to start your workout.

5. **Reward Yourself:** Set up a reward system for reaching milestones. Rewards can be anything from a new workout outfit to a relaxing massage.

6. **Create a Routine:** Consistency is vital. Try exercising at the same time every day to form a habit.

7. **Visualize Success:** Imagine yourself achieving your fitness goals. Visualization can be a powerful tool to maintain motivation.

1.3 Understanding Your Body's Changes

As we age, our bodies undergo a series of natural transformations that can affect our physical capabilities. Recognizing and understanding these changes helps us adapt our fitness routines to maintain our health and vitality. After age 50, one of the most significant changes is decreased muscle mass and bone density, known as sarcopenia and osteopenia. This gradual loss can lead to a weaker physique, reduced endurance, and a higher risk of fractures. Additionally, our metabolism slows down, contributing to weight gain and decreased energy levels, making it harder to stay active and manage weight through diet alone.

Strength training emerges as a powerful tool to counter these age-related declines. By engaging in regular resistance-based exercises, you can stimulate muscle growth, no matter your age. This not only helps increase muscle mass but also enhances bone density. Stronger muscles contribute to better balance and coordination, reducing the risk of falls, which is particularly important as bones become more fragile. Moreover, strength training can revitalize your metabolism, allowing your body to burn more calories—even at rest. This metabolic boost is essential in managing weight and maintaining energy levels, empowering you to lead an active and engaged life.

In this book, we will primarily focus on strength training. However, good exercise routines should include activities that improve heart health (aerobic exercises), build muscle strength (resistance exercises), increase flexibility (stretching), and improve balance (such as yoga). To that end, I have included some band exercises, alternatives to hand weights, and some yoga for beginning and ending your workouts.

The hormonal changes accompanying aging also significantly affect how our bodies react to physical stress and recovery. The most notable change for women is the decrease in estrogen levels due to menopause. This reduction in estrogen can lead to decreased muscle strength and recovery speed, making it harder to recover from injuries and fatigue. As we age, we might need more recovery time between workouts, focusing on lower-intensity or higher-repetition exercises or incorporating more flexibility and balance training to complement strength exercises.

Please don't get discouraged by fatigue after a workout; log it in your journal, give your body time to recover, and stay the course. Beyond the physical aspects, it's essential to consider the psychological impacts of aging. It's not uncommon to experience feelings of anxiety or depression as we move through later stages of life. However, regular physical activity, like strength training, improves mood and cognitive function. This improvement results from a release of endorphins, often called 'feel-good' hormones, which can naturally elevate your mood and combat stress. Additionally, the sense of achievement from meeting strength goals can boost your self-esteem and confidence, providing a significant mental uplift.

Given these complex physiological, hormonal, and psychological interactions, consult a healthcare provider before starting any new exercise regimen. A healthcare professional can offer valuable insights into tailoring your strength training program to your specific health conditions and needs. They can assess your health status and consider chronic conditions like arthritis or diabetes. All women should ask their doctor for a bone density scan if they have not recently had one.

Understanding how muscles grow can help with effective strength training. Muscles grow through a process involving motor neurons that signal muscle fibers to contract, creating muscle strength. This process is essential because, as we age, women naturally lose lean muscle due to factors like menopause. When women lift weights, the muscle fibers are repaired and increase in size during rest periods, leading to muscle growth. This growth is facilitated by satellite cells, which add new muscle fibers. Strength training doesn't make women bulky because they have less testosterone, but it helps them become more toned and stronger.

The growth of muscles is driven by three main mechanisms: muscle tension, muscle damage, and metabolic stress. Muscle tension occurs when lifting progressively heavier weights, causing changes in muscle chemistry that lead to growth. Muscle damage, felt as soreness after a workout activates satellite cells to repair and build muscle fibers. Metabolic stress, the "burn" during exercise, causes cell swelling and increases muscle size. These combined processes help build and maintain muscle.

Hormones also play a significant role in muscle growth for women. Chapter 3 reviews these hormones and their changes during midlife. Women have less testosterone than men, but strength training can increase hormone sensitivity and aid in muscle repair and growth. Muscle repair and growth happen during rest periods, not during the workout. While muscle growth can be slow, primarily due to genetic factors, consistent training, and proper nutrition help ensure that muscle protein synthesis exceeds breakdown, leading to visible muscle improvements over time.

1.4 Setting Up Your Home Gym with Minimal Equipment

Many people think you must join a gym or hire a personal trainer. Both are good options; having a trainer can help you learn the movements. However, starting neither option is necessary, especially if you are on a budget. This section will help you assemble an area in your home where you can begin this life-changing activity. You may also prefer working out in the comfort of your home, listening to the music you like, and having close access to your things—water, privacy, and bathroom. These are considerations that should not be discounted. Many find gyms distracting and intimidating and worry about using the machinery correctly. Thus, setting up a space at home may be the answer. Creating a practical and inviting home gym does not need to be expensive or require a lot of space. Let's discuss how you can start with just a few essential pieces of equipment, making the most of the area you have.

I recommend three core items for anyone starting their home gym: resistance bands, a yoga mat, and a set of dumbbells. These items are affordable and incredibly versatile, allowing you to perform various exercises targeting different muscle groups. Resistance bands, for instance, are fantastic for strength training, as they provide varying resistance levels and can be used for everything from bicep curls to leg extensions. A yoga mat provides a comfortable, stable surface for floor exercises and stretching. Dumbbells or kettlebells are perfect resistance workouts to build muscle strength and endurance.

Now, let's talk about setting up your space. Even if you're limited in area, you can still create an efficient workout zone. First, choose a space free of clutter and away from high-traffic areas in your home. Choose a corner of your bedroom, a part of your living room, or even a cleared-out area in your garage. The key is to have enough space to move freely in all directions. Good lighting is not only important for visibility but also essential in ensuring that you can maintain proper form during your exercises. I also like a wall mirror because I can see exactly what I'm doing. Additionally, consider the flooring—beyond the yoga mat, there are interlocking foam floor tiles that can provide a cushioned surface that is gentle on your joints and defines your workout space.

With these tips, your home gym will be ready quickly, providing you with a private, convenient spot to work on your fitness goals whenever suits you best. For example, my home gym is behind my sofa in the family room. I put down interlocking foam tiles to protect myself (and the floor). I have a used treadmill, a bench, and an adjustable set of dumbbells to give me much flexibility as my abilities change. Try starting with 5lb, 8lb, 10lb, 12lb dumbbells, and a few kettlebells. However, you can begin to smaller or bigger, depending on your current fitness level and budget for a home gym.

1.5 Tailoring Your Space for Safe Training

As you progress in your fitness journey, your needs might change, necessitating adjustments to your workout area. Have a flexible setup to modify as your strength and stamina increase. Adjustable dumbbells, for instance, are an excellent investment as they can be modified for different weights depending on your strength level and the type of exercise you are performing. Similarly, if you utilize resistance bands, having a variety of bands with different tension levels allows you to adjust the intensity of your workouts as you become stronger.

Adaptability makes your space more functional and aligns with your evolving fitness goals.

Create an inviting and comfortable training environment. Start with proper ventilation; ensure that your space is well-aired, which can help you stay relaxed and comfortable during workouts. Good airflow reduces the risk of overheating and helps keep the workout area fresh. Adequate lighting enhances safety by improving visibility and boosting your energy levels and mood. Consider setting up your workout area near natural light or invest in bright, warm artificial lighting. Add elements that inspire you, such as plants, or even play energizing music to make your space more personal and motivating. These personal touches can make your workout area a place where you enjoy spending time, which is essential for long-term adherence to any fitness regimen.

1.6 The First Step: Fitness Assessment

In your journal, write out where you are right now. Use the assessment tool below to start.

After conducting these assessments, set your baselines. Your current performance metrics serve as a starting point against which to measure progress. Write down your stats for each of these and revisit them after one month; you will be amazed at how quickly a regular, safe strength training and fitness routine will expand your fitness level. When you take the time to fill out the questionnaire, you can get clear on your goals, and you may be surprised at what you see for yourself!

Remember to document these in your fitness journal or a digital app (which we will discuss later) to keep track of improvements, no matter how small. This practice can be incredibly motivating. For instance, if you can initially do five chair squats without a break and, in a month, you can do ten, that's tangible progress! These baselines must be realistic and personalized—reflecting your fitness level and not an arbitrary standard. Check-in with your doctor, especially if you have current mobility considerations. This new venture will likely be applauded and encouraged!

Fitness Assessment Worksheet

Age: _____   Date: _____

Current Fitness Level

1. How often do you engage in physical activity?
Rarely / Occasionally / Regularly / Daily

2. What types of physical activities do you currently do?
(e.g., walking, yoga, swimming) - _____

3. On a scale of 1 to 10, how would you rate your overall fitness level?
(1 = Poor, 10 = Excellent) - _____

4. Do you experience shortness of breath during physical activities? - Yes / No

5. Do you feel pain or discomfort during or after physical activities? - Yes / No
If yes, please specify: _____

Fitness Goals

1. What are your primary fitness goals? (Check all that apply)

- ☐ Improve muscle strength
- ☐ Increase flexibility
- ☐ Improve balance
- ☐ Lose weight
- ☐ Enhance overall health
- ☐ Other: _____

2. How many times a week would you like to do strength training?

_____

3. Are there any specific areas you want to focus on? (e.g., arms, legs, core)

_____

Physical Assessments

1. Height: _____

2. Weight: _____

3. Body Measurements:

Waist: _____

Hips: _____

Chest: _____

Thigh: _____

Functional Movement Screen

1. Squat Test: How many bodyweight squats can you perform in 1 minute?

_____ (Use a chair or bench)

2. Push-up Test: How many push-ups can you perform in 1 minute?

_____ (Wall push-ups are acceptable)

3. Plank Test: How long can you hold a plank position?

_____ second(s) (Knees on the ground are okay)

4. Balance Test: How long can you stand on one leg without support?

_____ minute(s)

Squat Test

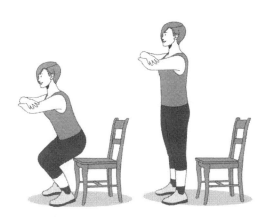

Proper Form:
- Keep your weight in your heels. This engages your glutes and prevents putting too much strain on your knees.
- Protect your lower back by avoiding rounding your back.
- Perform the squats in a slow and controlled manner to maximize muscle engagement and reduce the risk of injury.
- Inhale as you lower into the squat, and exhale as you rise back up.

Setup:
- Place a sturdy chair on a flat surface. You can also use a bench if that is part of your home gym.
- Stand in front of the chair with your feet hip-width apart.
- Position the chair so you can sit comfortably without moving your feet.

Starting Position:
- Stand tall with your shoulders back and your chest up.
- Extend your arms straight out in front of you for balance.
- Engage your core muscles to maintain a stable position.

Performing the Exercise:
- Push your hips back as if you are going to sit down in the chair.
- Bend your knees and lower your body toward the chair, keeping your chest up and your back straight.
- Make sure your knees are over your toes but not going past them.
- Lower yourself until your buttocks lightly touch the chair. Do not sit down fully.
- To rise, press through your heels and engage your glutes and thighs to stand back up. Keep your chest lifted and your core engaged.

Push-up Test

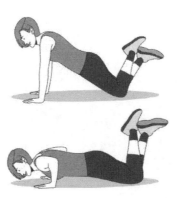

Proper Form:
- Keep your body straight from your head to your knees throughout the exercise. Avoid sagging your hips or arching your back.
- Perform each push-up in a slow and controlled manner.
- Inhale as you lower your body and exhale as you push back up.

Modified push-ups on your knees are an excellent way to build upper body strength while reducing the strain on your shoulders and lower back.

Setup:
- Begin by kneeling on a flat, comfortable surface. You may want to use a yoga mat or soft surface to cushion your knees.
- Place your hands on the ground slightly wider than shoulder-width apart. Your fingers should be pointing forward.

Starting Position:
- Shift your body weight forward so your shoulders are directly over your hands.
- With knees on the ground, lift your feet off the floor and cross your ankles.
- Your body should straighten from your head to your knees.
- Keep your head neutral by looking down at the floor.

Performing the Exercise:
- Inhale as you slowly lower your chest toward the ground; exhale as you rise.
- Bend your elbows, keeping them at a 45-degree angle to your body (not flaring out to the sides).
- Lower yourself until your chest is about an inch or two from the floor or as low as is comfortable for you. Don't worry if you can't get anywhere near the floor, keep it up and eventually you will see advancements.

Plank Test

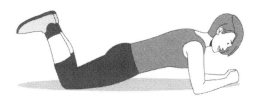

Proper Form
- Engage your core to maintain proper alignment and reduce strain on your lower back.
- Focus on steady, even breathing. Don't hold your breath.

Modified planks with knees down are a great way to build core strength and stability while reducing the strain on your lower back and shoulders.

Setup:
- Begin by kneeling on a flat, comfortable surface, like a yoga mat.
- Place your forearms on the ground directly below your shoulders, with your elbows bent at a 90-degree angle.

Starting Position:
- Extend your body so your knees, hips, and shoulders form a straight line.
- Keep your knees on the ground; position them slightly apart for stability.
- Your toes can either rest on the floor or lift off slightly, depending on your comfort.
- Engage your core muscles by pulling your belly button toward your spine.

Performing the Exercise:
- Hold this position for the desired amount of time, typically starting with 20-30 seconds and gradually increasing as you build strength.
- Ensure that your hips are neither sagging toward the floor nor lifting up too high. Maintain a straight line from your head to your knees.
- Engage your glutes and thighs to help stabilize your body.

Balance Test

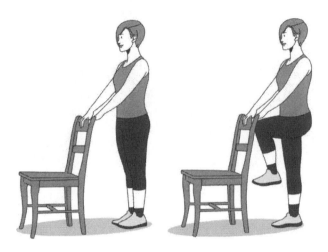

Performing a balance test can help assess your stability and coordination.

Setup:
- Find a flat, stable surface where you can stand safely.
- Stand near a wall or a sturdy piece of furniture for support, especially if you are new to balance exercises.

Starting Position:
- Stand with your feet hip-width apart and arms relaxed at your sides.
- Engage your core muscles to help maintain stability.

Performing the Exercise:
- Shift your weight onto your left foot and slowly lift your right foot off the ground.
- Bend your right knee, bringing your foot up behind you. Keep your raised knee facing forward, not turning it to the side.
- Hold this position for as long as possible, up to 30 seconds, while keeping your torso upright and steady.
- Try to maintain your balance without holding onto anything. If necessary, lightly touch the wall or furniture for support.
- Note the amount of time you can hold yourself on each leg.

Regular re-evaluation as your fitness level improves will show you what was challenging a few months ago has become easy, and your routines will need adjustment to remain beneficial. Reviewing and adjusting your exercise plan in consultation with fitness or health professionals who can provide guidance based on your progress and any new health considerations is good practice.

This ongoing assessment cycle, baseline setting, goal adaptation, and re-evaluation form a solid foundation for your strength training regimen. It ensures that your fitness activities evolve as you do, continually challenging you and meeting your body's changing needs. Remember, the ultimate goal is maintaining mobility, strength, and independence, enhancing your quality of life. Let these assessments guide you as you move forward, showing you where you need to go and how far you have come.

Let's get moving!

2

The Beginner's Strength Training Routine

Here is a weight training routine to consider if you are a beginner; it should not take more than 30 minutes, but don't rush; this is something positive you are doing for your health, so enjoy. Remember to warm up first. These poses help to gently stretch and warm up your muscles, increase blood flow, and prepare your body for the physical demands of strength training. Yoga is often used as a starting point for strength training, as it sets a strong foundation for your routine and helps you connect your mind and body.

Warm Up Routine:

Cat-Cow Pose (Marjaryasana-Bitilasana)

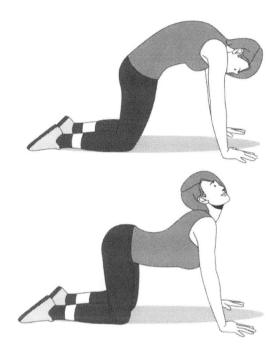

Cow Pose: Exhale and round your spine toward the ceiling, tucking your chin to your chest and drawing your belly in.

Cat Pose: Start on all fours with your wrists under your shoulders and knees under your hips. Inhale and arch your back, dropping your belly toward the mat. Lift your head and tailbone.

Repeat these movements, flowing with your breath.

Downward-Facing Dog (Adho Mukha Svanasana)

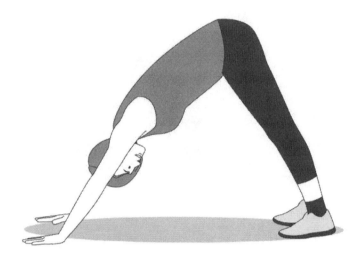

Start on all fours. Tuck your toes under and lift your hips toward the ceiling, straightening your legs and forming an inverted V-shape. Keep your hands shoulder-width apart and feet hip-width apart. Press your heels toward the floor and relax your head between your arms. This pose stretches the hamstrings, calves, and shoulders, preparing your body for more intense activity. Don't worry if you need to keep some bend in your knees or your heels are off the floor. We all have different flexibility limits, especially if you are starting.

Child's Pose (Balasana)

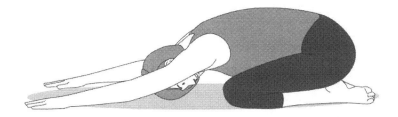

Kneel on the floor with your big toes touching and knees spread apart. Sit back on your heels and extend your arms forward, lowering your chest to the floor. Rest your forehead on the mat and breathe deeply. This pose helps to stretch the back, hips, and shoulders and provides a gentle way to ease into your workout. If this position is hard on your knees, then put a folded towel or yoga block/bolster under your hips. While you may not be as flexible as your goal, none of this should hurt.

Beginner Strength Training Weekly Workout Split

Build foundational strength and improve overall fitness. If you aren't doing any other fitness routines, you may want to start with just two days per week. Remember, the goal isn't perfection but getting moving in a way that supports your health and wellness habits. The warm-up, workout, and stretching should take approximately 30 minutes; take your time and enjoy seeing what your body can do.

Day 1: Full Body

Chair Squats (lower body)	3 sets of 10-12 reps
Wall Push-ups (upper body)	3 sets of 10-12 reps
Bent Over Dumbbell Rows (back)	3 sets of 8-10 reps
Dumbbell Shoulder Press (shoulders)	3 sets of 8-10 reps
Plank (core)	3 sets of 20-30 seconds

Day 2: Rest or Light Activity (e.g., walking, yoga)

Day 3: Full Body

Lunges (lower body)	3 sets of 10-12 reps (each leg)
Chest Press (chest)	3 sets of 8-10 reps
Bent Over Dumbbell Rows (back)	3 sets of 8-10 reps
Bicep Curls (arms)	3 sets of 10-12 reps
Plank (core)	3 sets of 40 seconds

Day 4: Rest or Light Activity

Day 5: Full Body

Glute Bridges (lower body)	3 sets of 10-12 reps
Lat Pulldown with Mini Bands (back)	3 sets of 10-12 reps
Dumbbell Flys (chest)	3 sets of 8-10 reps
Triceps Kickbacks (arms)	3 sets of 8-10 reps
Bird Dog (core/balance)	3 sets of 10-12 reps (each side)

Day 6: Rest or Light Activity

Day 7: Rest

Instructions for Each Exercise:

Chair Squats: (You can graduate to using weights when you are ready; I still use the bench/chair because it takes the guesswork out of whether I'm squatting low enough without going too low). Instructions are above in the assessment section.

Wall Push-ups: When you can easily do these sets/reps, you can graduate to floor push-ups or a modified version, like the one shown in the assessment section.

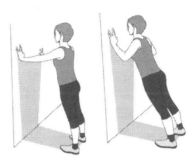

A wall push-up is an excellent beginner-friendly exercise that targets the chest, shoulders, and triceps. Here are the steps to perform a wall push-up correctly:

Setup:
- Stand facing a wall at arm's length.
- Place your hands on the wall at shoulder height and slightly wider than shoulder-width apart. Your fingers should point upward.

Starting Position:
- Keep your feet together or slightly apart for balance.
- Your body should be straight from head to heels, engaging your core muscles to maintain a neutral spine.

Performing the Exercise:
- Slowly bend your elbows and lower your chest toward the wall.
- Keep your elbows at a 45-degree angle relative to your body.
- Continue lowering until your nose or forehead is close to the wall.
- Push away from the wall, then return to the starting position.
- Ensure your body remains straight throughout the movement, avoiding sagging or arching your back.

Bent Over Rows

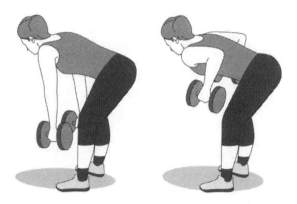

Bent-over rows are an excellent exercise for targeting the muscles in your back, including the latissimus dorsi, rhomboids, and trapezius, as well as your biceps and core. Here's how to perform them correctly:

Setup:
- Select a pair of dumbbells and stand with your feet shoulder-width apart. Mix and match with kettlebells to expand the variety of your workouts.
- Hold a dumbbell in each hand with a neutral grip (palms facing each other).
- Hinge at the hips to bend forward, keeping a slight bend in your knees. Your torso should be nearly parallel to the floor.
- Let your arms hang straight down from your shoulders.

Starting Position:
- Engage your core to maintain a neutral spine.
- Keep your head in line with your spine by looking at a spot on the floor a few feet before you.

Performing the Exercise:
- Exhale as you pull the dumbbells toward your lower ribcage, keeping your elbows close to your body.
- Squeeze your shoulder blades together at the top of the movement.
- Pause briefly at the top of the row to maximize muscle contraction.
- Inhale as you slowly lower the dumbbells back to the starting position, fully extending your arms.
- Maintain control of the weights throughout the movement.

Dumbbell Shoulder Press

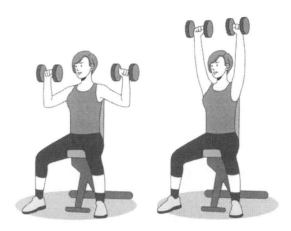

The dumbbell shoulder press is an effective exercise for building strength and muscle in your shoulders, specifically targeting the deltoids. It also engages your triceps and upper chest. Here's how to perform the dumbbell shoulder press correctly:

Setup:
- Select a pair of dumbbells of appropriate weight.
- Sit on a chair or bench with your feet shoulder-width apart. You can also perform this exercise sitting back in the chair for support.

Starting Position:
- Hold a dumbbell in each hand at shoulder height with your palms facing forward and your elbows bent at a 90-degree angle. Your upper arms should be parallel to the floor.
- Engage your core to maintain a stable and upright posture.

Performing the Exercise:
- Exhale as you press the dumbbells upward until your arms are fully extended above your head. Ensure your elbows are slightly bent at the top to avoid locking them out.
- Keep the weights moving in a straight line and avoid leaning back excessively.
- Inhale as you slowly lower the dumbbells back to the starting position at shoulder height.
- Maintain control of the weights throughout the movement.

Plank

Begin in a face-down position on the floor, propped up with your forearms and toes. Keep your body straight from your shoulders to your ankles, engaging your core to prevent your hips from sagging. Holding this position even for a few seconds can increase core strength and stability. Instructions are above in the assessment section.

Lunges

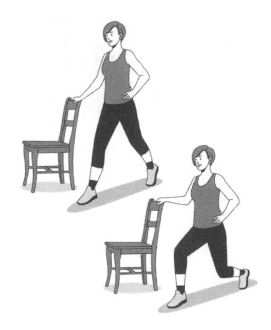

Setup:
- Grab a sturdy chair that won't slide or tip over when you apply pressure. If your balance is good, you can perform this move near a wall to give you a support option if needed.
- Ensure you have enough room around you to perform lunges safely.

Starting Position:
- Stand with your feet hip-width apart, holding onto the backrest of the chair with one hand for support. Keep your back straight and your shoulders relaxed.

Performing the Lunge:
- Take a step forward with your right foot, placing it firmly on the ground.
- Ensure your right knee is directly above your ankle and not extending beyond your toes.
- Slowly lower your body by bending both knees. Your back knee should move toward the ground, while your front knee stays aligned with your ankle.
- Keep your upper body straight and engage your core for stability.
- Push through the heel of your front foot to rise back up to the starting position.
- Bring your back foot forward to meet your front foot.

Chest Press with Dumbbells

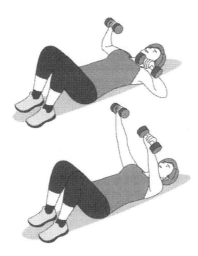

The chest press is a fundamental exercise that targets the chest muscles (pectorals), shoulders (deltoids), and triceps.

Dumbbell Chest Press

Setup:
- Select a pair of dumbbells of appropriate weight.
- Lie on the floor with your knees bent and feet flat on the ground or on a bench. Avoid arching your back too much.
- Hold a dumbbell in each hand, resting them on your thighs.

Starting Position:
- Use your thighs to help lift the dumbbells up, then position them directly above your chest with your palms facing forward.
- Bend your elbows at a 90-degree angle so your upper arms rest on the floor.

Performing the Exercise:
- Exhale as you press the dumbbells upward until your arms extend above your chest.
- Ensure your wrists are straight and your elbows are slightly bent at the top to avoid locking them out.
- Inhale as you slowly lower the dumbbells until your upper arms touch the floor again.
- Maintain control of the weights throughout the movement.

Bicep Curls

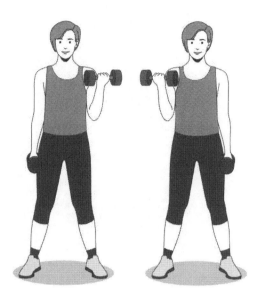

Dumbbell curls are an effective exercise to strengthen your biceps. Here's how to perform a standard dumbbell curl:

Setup:
- Stand with your feet shoulder-width apart, holding a dumbbell in each hand. Allow your arms to hang at your sides.

Performing the Exercise:
- Keep your upper arms to the elbows close to your sides and exhale as you curl the weights while contracting your biceps.
- Continue to raise the weights until your biceps are fully contracted and the dumbbells are at shoulder level. Hold the contracted position for a brief pause as you squeeze your biceps.
- Inhale as you slowly lower the dumbbells back to the starting position.

Bird Dog

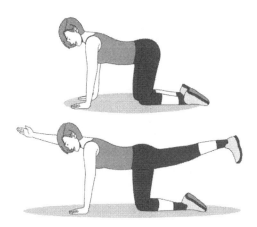

The bird dog exercise is an effective core stability exercise that targets the lower back, glutes, and abdominal muscles. It also helps improve balance and coordination. Here's how to perform the bird dog exercise correctly, along with some advanced options to increase the difficulty:

Setup:
- Begin on all fours with your hands directly under your shoulders and your knees directly under your hips.
- Engage your core muscles to keep your spine neutral. Your back should be flat, and your head should align with your spine.

Performing the Exercise:
- Extend your right arm before you while extending your left leg straight behind you.
- Keep your arm and leg parallel to the floor, with your fingers pointing forward and your toes pointing backward.
- Ensure your hips and shoulders remain square to the floor, avoiding rotation.
- Hold this extended position briefly (2-3 seconds) while maintaining balance and stability.
- Focus on keeping your core engaged and your body aligned.
- Slowly lower your right arm and left leg back to the starting position.
- Repeat the movement with your left arm and right leg.

Advanced Options for the Bird Dog:

Tips for Advanced Options:

- **Start with Light Resistance:** If using resistance bands or dumbbells, start with light resistance to avoid straining your muscles.

- **Maintain Form:** Focus on maintaining proper form and alignment, even with the added challenge.

- **Increase Gradually:** As your strength and stability improve, gradually increase the difficulty by adding resistance or balance challenges.

Bird Dog with Elbow to Knee Touch:

- **Setup:** Start in the standard bird dog position.

- **Performing the Exercise:** As you extend your right arm and left leg, bring them back in and touch your right elbow to your left knee under your body.

- **Extension:** Extend them back out to the starting position and repeat.

Glute Bridges

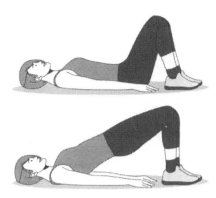

The glute bridge is a great exercise for strengthening the glutes, hamstrings, and lower back. It can also improve hip mobility and core stability.

Setup:
- Lie on your back on a flat, comfortable surface, such as a yoga mat.
- Bend your knees and place your feet flat on the ground, hip-width apart. Your heels should be about 6-8 inches away from your glutes.
- Rest your arms at your sides with your palms facing down.

Starting Position:
- Engage your core by drawing your belly button toward your spine.
- Press your lower back into the floor to eliminate any arch in your spine.

Performing the Exercise:
- Exhale as you lift your hips toward the ceiling. Press through your heels, squeezing your glutes at the top of the movement.
- Lift until your body forms a straight line from your shoulders to your knees. Your shoulders and upper back should remain in contact with the floor.
- Hold the position at the top for a moment, ensuring a strong glute contraction.
- Inhale as you slowly lower your hips back to the starting position.
- Maintain control throughout the descent, avoiding any sudden drops.

Dumbbell Flys

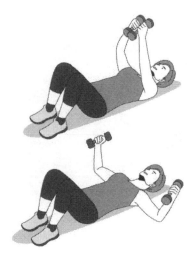

Dumbbell flys are effective for targeting the chest muscles (pectorals) and improving upper body strength.

Setup:
- Select a pair of dumbbells of appropriate weight.
- Lie flat on the floor with your feet flat on the ground. Your head, shoulders, and glutes should be in contact with the floor.
- Hold a dumbbell in each hand with your arms extended straight up above your chest, palms facing each other. Your elbows should have a slight bend to reduce stress on the joints.

Starting Position:
- Engage your core to maintain a stable and upright posture.
- Keep your shoulders down and back, pressing them against the floor or bench.

Performing the Exercise:
- Inhale as you slowly lower the dumbbells out to the sides in a wide arc, maintaining the slight bend in your elbows. Lower the weights until they are level with your chest or slightly above it, feeling a stretch in your chest muscles.
- Ensure that your elbows remain in line with your shoulders and do not drop too low to avoid unnecessary strain.
- Exhale as you bring the dumbbells back up to the starting position, following the same wide arc. Squeeze your chest muscles at the top of the movement.
- Ensure that the movement is controlled and that you are not using momentum.

Resistance Band Lat Pulldowns

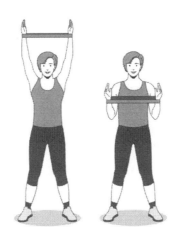

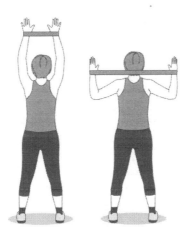

The lat pulldown exercise with a mini band is an excellent way to target the latissimus dorsi muscles (lats) in your back, biceps, and shoulders. Using the mini band is great because you don't need the machinery found in gyms to get a great result.

You can pull the band to the front or the back. Here, you need to be mindful of your shoulders—the back version is harder on mine. I always pull down to the front, but everyone's flexibility varies. Try the movement with no band first to see how your shoulders feel.

Lat Pulldown to the Front with a Mini Band

Setup:
- Select a mini band with appropriate resistance.
- Sit or stand with your feet shoulder-width apart.
- Hold the mini band with both hands, gripping it slightly wider than shoulder-width apart.
- Extend your arms above your head, keeping tension in the band.

Starting Position:
- Engage your core to maintain an upright posture.
- Keep your shoulders relaxed and away from your ears.

Performing the Exercise:
- Exhale as you pull the mini band down toward your chest, bending your elbows and squeezing your shoulder blades together.
- Continue pulling until your elbows are in line with your shoulders and the band is just above or touching your chest.
- Focus on using your back muscles to perform the movement, not just your arms.
- Inhale as you slowly return to the starting position, extending your arms overhead while maintaining tension in the band.
- Control the movement to avoid snapping the band back.

Lat Pulldown to the Back with a Mini Band

Setup:
- Follow the same setup as for the front pulldown.
- Sit or stand with your feet shoulder-width apart.
- Hold the mini band with both hands, gripping it slightly wider than shoulder-width apart.
- Extend your arms above your head, keeping tension in the band.

Starting Position:
- Engage your core to maintain an upright posture.
- Keep your shoulders relaxed and away from your ears.

Performing the Exercise:
- Exhale as you pull the mini band down toward the back of your neck, bending your elbows and squeezing your shoulder blades together.
- Continue pulling until your elbows align with your shoulders and the band is just behind your head.
- Focus on using your back muscles to perform the movement, not just your arms.
- Inhale as you slowly return to the starting position, extending your arms overhead while maintaining tension in the band.
- Control the movement to avoid snapping the band back.

Triceps Kickbacks

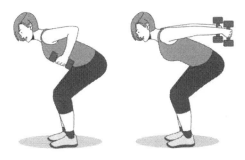

Triceps kickbacks are an excellent exercise for targeting the triceps, the muscles at the back of your upper arms.

Setup:
- Select a pair of dumbbells with an appropriate weight.
- Stand with your feet shoulder-width apart and hold a dumbbell in each hand.
- Bend your knees slightly and hinge forward at the hips until your torso is nearly parallel to the floor. Keep your back straight and your core engaged.

Starting Position:
- Bend your elbows to 90 degrees, bringing the dumbbells up to your sides. Your upper arms should be parallel to the floor.
- Keep your head neutral by looking down at the floor.

Performing the Exercise:
- Exhale as you extend your arms straight back, keeping your upper arms stationary. Only your forearms should move.
- Squeeze your triceps at the top of the movement and hold briefly.
- Inhale as you slowly bring the dumbbells back to the starting position with your elbows bent at 90 degrees.
- Maintain control throughout the movement.

Resistance Bands and Kettlebells

Resistance bands are versatile exercise tools that come in various types, each designed for different levels of resistance and types of exercises. Here are the main types of resistance bands:

Loop Bands (Mini Bands) are small, flat loops typically made of rubber or latex. They're commonly used for lower body exercises like glute bridges, lateral walks, and squats and are great for targeting smaller muscle groups.

Therapy Bands (Flat Bands) are flat, non-looped bands, often made of latex or rubber, available in long strips. They are used for stretching and are great for upper-body exercises.

Tube Bands with Handles are round, tube-shaped bands with handles on each end. These bands are great for full-body workouts, particularly upper-body exercises like bicep curls, shoulder presses, and rows. The handles provide a firm grip, making them versatile and easy to use.

Figure 8 Bands are shaped like a figure 8 with two handles, one at each loop. They are commonly used for upper body exercises, especially for targeting the chest, shoulders, and arms.

Here are some examples that you can incorporate into your workouts for variety.

Two variations on leg extensions and an option for the bent-over row:

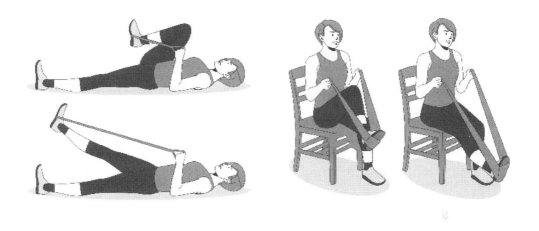

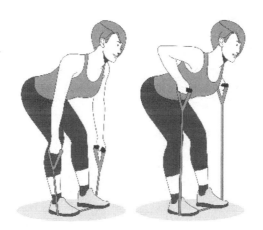

Benefits of Kettlebells:

Kettlebells offer several unique benefits compared to traditional hand weights (dumbbells), bringing distinct advantages to strength training and fitness routines.

Full-Body Workouts: Kettlebell exercises typically involve compound movements, engaging multiple muscle groups simultaneously. This leads to a more comprehensive full-body workout that improves strength, endurance, and cardiovascular fitness.

Functional Strength: Kettlebell training emphasizes functional movements that mimic everyday activities, such as lifting, carrying, and swinging. This can enhance your ability to perform daily tasks more efficiently and reduce the risk of injury.

Improved Core Stability: The off-centered weight of kettlebells requires you to engage your core more actively to maintain balance and control during exercises. This leads to better core stability and strength.

Enhanced Coordination and Balance: The dynamic nature of kettlebell exercises, such as swings and snatches, challenges coordination and balance, which can lead to improved overall body control and proprioception.

Versatility: Kettlebells can be used for various exercises, from swings and snatches to squats and presses. They are also excellent for high-intensity interval training (HIIT), which can improve cardiovascular fitness and burn calories effectively.

Why Choose Kettlebells over Dumbbells:

Weight Distribution: The primary difference is in the weight distribution. A kettlebell's center of mass is several inches outside your grip, which challenges your stabilizing muscles more than a dumbbell, where the weight is evenly distributed on either side of the handle.

Grip and Handling: A kettlebell's handle is thicker and usually wider than a dumbbell's, which can improve grip strength. The design also allows for more fluid, swinging motions, which are not typically performed with dumbbells.

Exercise Variety: While dumbbells are more straightforward and are often used for isolated muscle exercises, kettlebells are more suited to ballistic, dynamic movements. Exercises like the kettlebell swing or Turkish get-up are unique to kettlebells and offer a different kind of challenge than what can be achieved with dumbbells. As your training advances, these could be a great addition to your routine.

Training Focus: Kettlebells are excellent for developing explosive power and functional strength and improving cardiovascular fitness. Dumbbells, however, are often used to focus on muscle hypertrophy (muscle growth) through more controlled, isolated movements.

Learning Curve: Kettlebell exercises often require more technique and practice to perform correctly, especially dynamic movements like swings, cleans, and snatches. Due to their simplicity, dumbbells are generally more manageable for beginners.

See the kettlebell variations under the Advanced

Summary:

Remember to start with a proper warm-up before each workout and finish with a cool-down and stretching. Adjust weights and repetitions as needed based on your fitness level and progress. Always consult a healthcare professional or fitness trainer before starting any new exercise program.

Choose your starting weight by testing out what weight you can lift twelve times, with the last few repetitions being more difficult than the first few. If you can keep lifting that weight with little effort each day, then you aren't doing yourself any good. You can always go lighter if you start heavier, and vice versa.

Building a routine in the initial weeks will establish a habit and set the stage for consistent progress. Start with two to three days per week, dedicating about 20 to 30 minutes per session. This frequency ensures that you are active enough to begin seeing improvements but also provides ample recovery time, which is critical as your muscles adjust to new activities.

Log your exercises and details in your journal. If you prefer, numerous apps can help you track your workouts. These digital tools often offer additional features like reminders, motivational quotes, and instructional videos, which can be incredibly helpful as you build and refine your workout regimen.

Consistency is vital in any fitness regimen but essential when starting. Regular exercise sessions help to form habits, making it easier to stick with your program long-term. Be sure to set realistic goals and gradually increase the intensity and duration of your workouts. This approach helps to prevent injuries and ensures steady progress. Remember, small, consistent steps lead to lasting changes. By gradually increasing the complexity and intensity of your workouts, you ensure that your fitness journey is sustainable and adapted to your evolving capabilities and goals.

Listen to your body and adjust your activities according to how you feel. Consider using lightweight bands that are great for traveling and kettlebells that are great for more advanced training. Modifying the exercise or even taking a rest day may be wise if you ever feel undue pain or discomfort.

3

Exercise Modifications

Don't let specific health conditions like arthritis stop your journey. After discussing a new regime with your doctor, consider that strength training doesn't have to be a strenuous ordeal. This chapter will guide you through selecting low-impact strength training exercises, managing exercise-related pain, and making necessary modifications on tough days. Together, we'll turn these challenges into a structured plan that respects your body's limits and celebrates its capabilities.

3.1 Low-impact Strength Training: Safe for Arthritis

Arthritis can make exercise more than a little daunting. Exercise is known to be an essential treatment for arthritis. However, over 40% of adults with arthritis say they don't do any physical activities in their free time. Incorporating gentle, joint-friendly exercises into your routine can significantly improve your strength and flexibility without overtaxing your body.

Activities like swimming and resistance band workouts stand out as ideal choices. With its buoyant support, swimming alleviates the impact on your joints while providing a comprehensive workout that enhances cardiovascular health and muscular endurance. It's like hugging your body while you exercise—the water's embrace takes the load off your joints, allowing you to move more freely and with less pain. There are also water weights so that you can do resistance training in the pool.

Resistance bands help build strength without heavy weights, which can be harsh on sensitive joints. By varying the tension and adjusting your stance, you can target different muscle groups with minimal risk. For instance, a seated band row can be performed by anchoring the band at a low point (like a door handle), sitting on a chair some distance away, and pulling the bands toward you. This exercise strengthens the back, shoulders, and arms, all crucial for improving your functional movement without any jarring impacts.

An effective strategy for managing pre-existing pain is applying heat or cold therapy before and after workouts. Warm up your joints with a heating pad to increase blood flow and flexibility before you start. Applying a cold pack can reduce inflammation and help manage pain. Remember, listen to your body and start slow. Begin with low-intensity sessions and gradually increase the duration and frequency as your body adapts. This careful, measured approach helps prevent overexertion and minimizes discomfort, making your workouts more enjoyable and effective.

On days when your symptoms flare up, modify your routine to accommodate your body's needs. Reducing the range of motion in exercises can help manage pain while still allowing you to stay active. For example, if a full squat is too painful, try performing a half-squat or using a chair to support some of your weight. Switching to lighter weights or using just your body weight can also reduce strain on your joints while still providing the benefits of resistance training. These modifications ensure you can continue working out, even on your most challenging days, helping you maintain consistency in your fitness regimen.

Furthermore, consulting with professionals like physical therapists or exercise physiologists can provide you with personalized advice and modifications. These experts can assess your needs and develop a tailored exercise plan that maximizes safety and effectiveness. They can also teach you how to perform exercises and use equipment to avoid injuries correctly. This professional guidance is invaluable, as it ensures that your health requirements are met, providing peace of mind and fostering better results from your workout efforts.

By embracing these low-impact exercises and pain management strategies and seeking professional guidance, you can create a workout regimen that strengthens your body without stressing your joints. This approach improves your physical health and enhances your quality of life, allowing you to stay active and enjoy your daily activities with fewer limitations. Remember, every movement counts, and with the proper modifications, you can achieve your fitness goals while taking good care of your joints.

3.2 Exercises to Enhance Bone Density Post-menopause

After menopause, many women notice changes in their metabolism and mood and a significant decrease in bone density. This natural decrease in bone strength is due to lower estrogen levels, which affect bone calcium and other mineral levels. However, the right exercises can significantly mitigate these effects. Weight-bearing exercises, resistance training, and certain impact activities are recommended to keep bones robust and healthy.

Weight-bearing exercises are your first line of defense against bone density loss. They make you move against gravity while staying upright, helping build bones and muscles. Walking is the simplest form of weight-bearing exercise, though it is one of the most effective. Whether a brisk walk in your neighborhood or using a treadmill, weight-bearing exercises are your first defense against bone density loss. They make you move against gravity while staying upright, helping build bones and muscles.

Strength training done correctly stresses your bones, encouraging the bone-forming cells to go into overdrive and increase bone mass. Start with lighter weights, and as you grow comfortable, you can gradually increase the resistance. It's vital to focus on form to prevent any strain or injury. For instance, when doing squats, ensure your back is straight and that you lower yourself as if you are going to sit in a chair, which helps keep the pressure on your legs rather than your back.

3.3 Adapting Workouts for Reduced Mobility

When mobility becomes limited due to age or injury, it doesn't mean the end of your ability to exercise and strengthen your body. Adapting your workout to fit your mobility level helps maintain your physical health and boosts your mental well-being by keeping you active and engaged. Let's explore how you can modify strength training exercises through seated and supported positions, utilize helpful assistive devices, customize routines to your needs, and incorporate regular movement into your daily life.

Seated and supported exercises are fantastic options for engaging in strength training without putting undue stress on your legs. For instance, you can perform upper body exercises such as shoulder presses, bicep curls, and lateral raises while seated comfortably in a chair. This position helps maintain stability and reduces the risk of falls, making exercise safer without impeding its effectiveness. Similarly, leg exercises can also be adapted to a seated position. Seated leg lifts, for example, can strengthen your thigh and abdominal muscles without requiring you to stand. By sitting down, you focus the effort on your upper body, keeping your spine straight and supported, which is excellent for those with back issues or reduced lower body strength.

Incorporating assistive devices into your workout routine can enhance your ability to perform exercises safely. A simple chair, for example, can offer stability and support during seated or standing exercises. Elastic bands are exceptionally versatile, and you can use them for various exercises that target both upper and lower body muscles. Using these tools, you can maintain proper exercise form and reduce the risk of strain or injury, making your workout experience both safe and enjoyable.

Customizing exercise routines to accommodate mobility limitations ensures you receive full-body benefits from your workouts. Start by assessing which movements are comfortable for you and build your routine around those. For instance, if bending your knees is challenging, focus on exercises that strengthen your upper body and core or use a pool to perform water aerobics, which minimizes joint stress. It's also helpful to break your workouts into shorter, more frequent sessions throughout the day if endurance is an issue. This method helps maintain energy levels and prevents fatigue while allowing you to achieve the cumulative effect of a complete workout. Consulting with a physical therapist or a fitness professional specializing in fitness for women as they age can provide personalized advice and adjustments, ensuring that each exercise effectively contributes to your strength without exceeding your limitations.

Lastly, incorporating movement throughout your day cannot be overstated. Regular movement helps maintain flexibility, prevents stiffness, and supports circulation—all vital for mobility. Simple activities like stretching your arms overhead, rotating your ankles while sitting, or standing up and sitting down a few times can significantly contribute to your mobility and overall health. Try setting reminders to move a little every hour or integrate these movements into your daily routines, such as doing arm stretches while watching TV or leg lifts while reading. These small actions can make a big difference in how you feel and function daily.

3.4 Strength Training with Osteoporosis: A Detailed Guide

Osteoporosis might sound like a roadblock to active living, but with the right approach to strength training, you can still enjoy the vast benefits of exercise while taking good care of your bones. Crafting a workout that respects the fragility of osteoporotic bones means prioritizing safety and effectiveness. Let's start this exploration by focusing on safe exercise practices specifically beneficial for individuals with osteoporosis.

Osteoporosis causes your bones to be more susceptible to fractures, so high-impact exercises can be more risky than beneficial. Instead, the emphasis should be on slow, controlled movements that enhance strength without undue stress. For instance, exercises using body weight, light weights, or resistance bands are ideal because they allow for controlled pressure that strengthens bones without the jarring impact that can cause damage. Activities like Pilates and yoga are also excellent, focusing on balance and muscle strengthening with a high degree of control. Moreover, maintaining a straight, strong posture during these exercises helps promote bone health, particularly in the spine.

Identifying and avoiding specific exercises that involve twisting your spine or bending forward from the waist can increase the risk of spine fractures and should be avoided. Traditional sit-ups and toe touches are examples of movements that can be harmful due to the spinal flexion they involve. Similarly, high-impact sports like running or jumping might be too harsh on your bones despite their general health benefits. Replacing these with low-impact, bone-strengthening exercises such as walking or elliptical training can offer a safer alternative, providing the stimulus your bones need to maintain their strength without the risky impact.

Building a safe routine starts with understanding these rules and integrating them into a coherent workout plan. Begin with a warm-up using gentle stretching to increase your muscle and joint flexibility, preparing them for exercise without strain. Incorporate strength training exercises targeting all major muscle groups, focusing on stability and muscle endurance rather than lifting heavy weights. For example, using resistance bands for a chest press instead of a bench press can reduce the risk to your spinal column while still fortifying chest, arm, and shoulder muscles. Aim to include balance exercises in every session since improving balance can significantly reduce the risk of falls. Exercises like the single-leg stand or using a balance board can be very effective.

Incorporating these principles into your strength training routine creates a safe environment to maintain physical health and enhance bone density. Remember, each exercise session is a step toward stronger bones and a more vibrant life, even with osteoporosis. By focusing on safe practices, avoiding risky exercises, building a thoughtful routine, and working closely with healthcare professionals, you can effectively manage your condition and enjoy the myriad benefits of strength training.

3.5 Building Core Strength for Better Balance and Stability

The core of your body is like the central support structure of a building. If it's solid and stable, it supports everything else—an essential factor as we age. Strengthening your core can significantly improve your balance and stability, reducing the risk of falls and other injuries. Let's dive into some exercises that are particularly beneficial for enhancing your core's strength, integrating balance training, and understanding the progressive levels of difficulty that can help you grow more robust and stable. In each weight-lifting exercise, the core should be engaged and spine neutral.

1. Engage Your Core:

- **Belly Button to Spine:** Imagine pulling your belly button towards your spine. This action engages the transverse abdominis, the deepest layer of your abdominal muscles, providing stability to your lower back.

- **Brace:** Think about bracing your core as if you're about to be punched in the stomach. This doesn't mean sucking in your stomach but rather tightening your abdominal muscles.

- **Breathing:** Maintain steady breathing. It's common to hold your breath when engaging your core, but try to breathe through it, especially when lifting weights.

2. Maintain a Neutral Spine:

- **Natural Curves:** Your spine has a natural S-curve, with a slight inward curve in your lower back and a slight outward curve in your upper back. Maintaining this curvature is essential to keep your back neutral.

- **Head Alignment:** Keep your head in line with your spine. Depending on the exercise, your gaze should be forward or slightly downward to avoid excessive strain on your neck.

- **Shoulder Position:** Pull your shoulders down and back. This helps maintain a neutral spine and prevents rounding of the upper back.

3. Hips and Pelvis:

- **Pelvic Tilt:** Avoid excessive pelvic tilting. Neither an excessive arch in the lower back (anterior pelvic tilt) nor tucking the tailbone under (posterior pelvic tilt) is ideal. Aim for a position where your pelvis is neutral and aligns with the natural curve of your spine.

- **Glute Engagement:** Engage your glutes to help stabilize your pelvis, especially during lower-body exercises like squats and deadlifts.

An exercise to strengthen your core is the pelvic tilt, which benefits the lower abdominal muscles and lower back while creating good posture and balance. Lie on your back with your knees bent and feet flat on the floor. Tighten your abdominal muscles and gently tilt your hips upward, flattening your back against the floor. Hold for a few seconds, then relax. This subtle movement fortifies the lower spine and abdominal area, enhancing core stability.

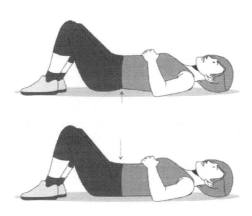

Pelvic Tilt

Purpose: The pelvic tilt exercise helps strengthen the abdominal muscles and lower back, improve posture, and reduce lower back pain.

Starting Position:

- Begin by lying on your back on a comfortable, flat surface. Bend your knees and place your feet flat, hip-width apart.
- Place your arms at your sides with your palms facing down.

Steps to Perform the Pelvic Tilt:

- Start by finding your neutral spine position. Your back should have a natural curve, with a small space between your lower back and the floor.
- Take a deep breath through your nose, allowing your abdomen to rise.
- As you exhale, gently flatten your lower back against the floor by tightening your abdominal muscles. This will cause your pelvis to tilt slightly upward.
- Hold this position for a few seconds while continuing to breathe normally. You should feel a gentle stretch in your lower back and a contraction in your abdominal muscles.
- Slowly release the tilt and return to the neutral spine as you inhale.

Repetitions:

- Perform 10-15 repetitions of the pelvic tilt.
- Rest for a few seconds between each repetition.

Modifications:

- **Advanced:** For an added challenge, try performing the pelvic tilt with one leg lifted off the ground.
- **Beginner:** If lying on the floor is uncomfortable, you can move similarly while standing against a wall.

3.6 Customizing Workouts: When and How to Modify Exercises

Understanding how to tailor your workout routine to meet your needs can dramatically enhance your exercise regimen's effectiveness and enjoyment. Develop the ability to listen to your body and recognize the signs that an exercise might need to be modified. This intuition can help you avoid discomfort and prevent potential injuries, ensuring a sustainable and beneficial workout experience. For instance, if you notice a sharp pain during a particular movement, it's a clear indicator that you should stop and adjust. Similarly, if you cannot maintain proper form—perhaps you're swaying during a lift or can't reach a full range of motion—it's time to consider modifying the exercise to suit your current level better.

Adapting exercises can be simple yet significantly effective in enhancing comfort and efficiency. Let's take the example of squats, a fundamental strength-training exercise. If a standard squat causes discomfort in your knees or you find it challenging to maintain balance, you can modify it using a chair. Perform a chair squat by starting in a seated position, standing up with weight evenly distributed on your feet, and then sitting back down with controlled motion. This modification reduces the strain on your knees and back while effectively engaging the core and lower body muscles. Another common modification is for the push-up. If a standard floor push-up is too challenging, you can begin by performing them against a wall or on an elevated surface like a bench to reduce the load on your arms and shoulders until you build more strength.

Utilizing props is another effective way to modify exercises to accommodate your physical capabilities and enhance the safety and effectiveness of your workout. Props such as blocks, straps, and cushions can significantly aid in achieving proper alignment and reducing strain. For example, if reaching the floor is difficult during a forward bend, placing a yoga block under your hands can bring the ground closer to you, allowing you to maintain the integrity of the pose without overstretching. Similarly, a strap can be helpful in a leg stretch by providing a way to hold your leg extended without straining your back or shoulders. Cushions or folded towels can give extra padding for knees or elbows during exercises requiring pressure on these joints, ensuring comfort and preventing pain.

As we wrap up this chapter on customizing workouts and modifying exercises, remember the key takeaways: listen to your body, use modifications to enhance comfort, employ props for support, and make dynamic adjustments as your fitness evolves. These strategies are essential in crafting a workout that respects your body's needs and efficiently pushes you toward your fitness goals. Next, we will explore advanced techniques and strategies to enhance your strength training regimen, ensuring you continue progressing and enjoying your fitness journey.

4

Nutrition, Recovery, and Weight Loss

Embarking on a strength training regimen during midlife is not just about the exercises you do—it's equally about fueling your body correctly. Think of your body as a finely-tuned vehicle that needs the right fuel to run efficiently and recover from the demands of each workout. This chapter will guide you through the nutritional essentials that support muscle recovery, which is vital for sustaining your strength training efforts and enhancing your overall health.

4.1 Nutrition Essentials: Eating for Muscle Recovery

Understanding the basics of a balanced diet is fundamental in supporting your body through strength training. Proteins, carbohydrates, and healthy fats play pivotal roles in muscle recovery. Proteins are the heroes here, serving as the building blocks of muscle repair and growth. After a workout, your muscles are eager for protein to help repair the micro-tears caused by lifting weights. Including a good protein source in your diet, such as chicken, fish, tofu, or beans, is a must for muscle recovery and growth.

Carbohydrates are often misunderstood, but they are also needed because they replenish the glycogen stores your body depletes during exercise. Whole grains, fruits, and vegetables are excellent sources of healthy carbohydrates that provide the energy you need for recovery and the next workout. Healthy fats, like those found in avocados, nuts, and olive oil, are vital for long-term energy storage and help your body absorb essential nutrients.

Timing your meals can also significantly impact how effectively your body recovers from exercise. Eating a snack or meal rich in protein and carbohydrates within 45 minutes to an hour after your workout can drastically improve muscle recovery. This window is when your muscles are most receptive to the nutrients that aid repair and growth. A simple post-workout snack could be a Greek yogurt with berries, a slice of whole-grain bread with peanut butter, or a small smoothie made with fruits and protein powder.

Timing

- **Within 30-60 Minutes After Workout**: Aim to eat a balanced meal or snack within this window for optimal recovery.

What to Eat

1. **Protein**: Essential for muscle repair and growth.
   - Examples: Lean meats (chicken, turkey), fish, eggs, dairy products (Greek yogurt, cottage cheese), plant-based options (tofu, tempeh, legumes), protein shakes

2. **Carbohydrates**: Replenish glycogen stores depleted during exercise.
   - Examples: Whole grains (brown rice, quinoa, whole grain bread), fruits (berries, bananas, apples), starchy vegetables (sweet potatoes, butternut squash)

3. **Healthy Fats**: Support overall health and can be included in moderation.
   - Examples: Avocado, nuts and seeds, olive oil, fatty fish (salmon, mackerel)

Post-workout Meal Ideas

- Grilled chicken with quinoa and steamed vegetables
- A smoothie made with protein powder, a banana, spinach, and almond milk
- A turkey and avocado whole-grain wrap
- Greek yogurt with a handful of mixed berries and a drizzle of honey
- A salad with mixed greens, grilled salmon, chickpeas, and a vinaigrette dressing

To help you integrate these nutritional principles into your daily routine, here are a few ideas that are nutritious and easy to prepare. Consider starting your day with an omelet packed with vegetables and a slice of whole-grain toast. For lunch, a quinoa salad with cherry tomatoes, cucumbers, feta cheese, and a drizzle of olive oil provides a balanced mix of protein, carbs, and fats. Dinner could be grilled salmon with sweet potato and steamed broccoli, which is ideal for muscle repair and is rich in micronutrients. These meals are simple and designed to make healthy eating a stress-free part of your daily life.

As your body ages, its nutritional needs change, and being over 50 means you need more protein than younger individuals to help maintain muscle mass and strength. Remember that building muscle in midlife requires weight training and consuming enough protein within the two-hour window after weight training. How much is enough? Many experts say at least 30 grams. It's also important to focus on calcium and vitamin D, both needed for bone health and significant concern for women post-menopausal. Dairy products, green leafy vegetables, and fortified foods can help meet these needs. Remember, the goal is to eat healthily and strategically to support your strength training and overall well-being.

Time to Journal

Be sure to journal the nutritious meals you prepare. Not only will this help you track your intake of proteins, carbs, and fats, but over time, this journal can serve as a motivational tool, showcasing the direct correlation between your diet, workouts, and overall feelings.

Pre-workout Snack Ideas

If you think having a snack before workouts is needed for energy or your doctor has suggested such, then having a small snack 30 to 60 minutes before a workout is a good idea. Consider these:

- A banana with a tablespoon of almond butter
- Greek yogurt with a handful of berries
- A slice of whole-grain toast with avocado
- A small smoothie made with spinach, a banana, and a scoop of protein powder
- A handful of nuts and an apple

Understanding and implementing these nutritional essentials can significantly enhance your body's ability to recover from workouts, maintain muscle mass, and improve overall energy and health. Remember, what you feed your body after a workout is as important as the workout itself. With the proper nutrients, you're not only replenishing what you've lost but also preparing your body for the challenges ahead, ensuring that you can continue to train effectively and see the results of your hard work.

4.2 The Role of Hydration in Effective Strength Training

Electrolytes, such as sodium, potassium, magnesium, and calcium, play a role in maintaining your body's hydration, nerve transmissions, and muscle function. When you sweat, not only do you lose water, but you also lose these essential minerals. Eating a well-balanced diet for most daily training sessions will provide you with the necessary electrolytes. However, you might need an extra boost if you engage in prolonged or intense workouts or sweat heavily. In such cases, incorporating an electrolyte drink can be beneficial. These drinks can help replenish your electrolyte balance more efficiently than water alone and provide a quick energy source to help you recover from your workout.

Approximately 65% of the total water in your body is inside your cells; the remainder is extracellular fluid or outside your cells. This means that as you age and lose muscle, you are also losing water. Weight training can help with this water loss. Without muscles to "hold" the reserve of water in your body, dehydration can occur more readily.

The signs of dehydration can be more subtle in older adults. Common signs include dry mouth, fatigue, dizziness, and darker-colored urine. If you experience these symptoms, they may be a signal from your body to increase your fluid intake. To prevent dehydration, make it a habit to carry a water bottle with you throughout the day. Set reminders on your phone or keep a hydration tracker handy to help you remember to take sips regularly, ensuring you are well-hydrated before you even lace up your sneakers.

Like all things, too much water isn't good either. Drinking too much water, also known as overhydration, can lead to hyponatremia, where the balance of electrolytes in your body is disrupted. The standard color of urine should be pale yellow to amber for a person drinking the right amount of water. This color range indicates proper hydration and a healthy balance of electrolytes and other substances in the urine.

In terms of frequency, a healthy person should urinate about 6-8 times a day. However, this can vary depending on fluid intake, age, medication use, and overall health. Urinating more frequently, particularly if accompanied by obvious urine, might indicate that you are drinking more water than necessary. Consulting a healthcare professional is always a good idea if you have concerns about your hydration status.

4.3 Supplements: What Helps and What Doesn't?

There are countless options and paths, but not all lead to better health. As a woman over 50, your body has specific nutritional requirements, especially when engaging in strength training. When used correctly, supplements can support your muscle recovery and overall health. However, caution is needed as not all supplements are beneficial, and some can even be detrimental.

Protein powders are among the most beneficial supplements for anyone in strength training. Protein is essential for muscle repair and growth, and while it's best to get most of your protein from whole foods, powders can be a convenient and efficient way to meet your daily needs, especially on busy days or when you need a quick recovery boost after a workout. Whey protein is popular due to its complete amino acid profile and fast absorption rate. However, if you are lactose intolerant or following a plant-based diet, options like pea or soy are excellent alternatives.

Omega-3 fatty acids are another supplement worth considering. Commonly found in fish oil capsules, they are known for their anti-inflammatory properties, which can help reduce muscle soreness and speed up recovery. Omega-3s also support heart health, joint mobility, and cognitive function—all crucial for maintaining an active lifestyle as you age.

They can also be found in various foods, including:

1. **Fatty Fish**:
   o Salmon
   o Mackerel
   o Sardines
   o Herring
   o Trout
   o Albacore tuna

2. **Seeds**:
   - Chia seeds
   - Flaxseeds (ground flaxseeds are easier to digest)
   - Hemp seeds
3. **Nuts**:
   - Walnuts
4. **Plant Oils**:
   - Flaxseed oil
   - Canola oil
   - Soybean oil
   - Walnut oil
5. **Seaweed and Algae**:
   - Nori (used in sushi)
   - Spirulina
   - Chlorella
6. **Fortified Foods**:
   - Omega-3 fortified eggs
   - Milk
   - Yogurt
   - Juice
7. **Vegetables**:
   - Brussels sprouts
   - Spinach
   - Kale

Vitamin D supplements can also be particularly beneficial, especially for women over 50. Vitamin D not only aids in calcium absorption, which is essential for bone health but also plays a role in muscle function. Since many individuals do not get sufficient vitamin D from sunlight, especially in colder climates, supplementation can be a critical factor in maintaining muscle health and overall well-being.

While these supplements can be beneficial, be wary of products that promise miraculous results. Supplements claiming to enhance strength or muscle mass drastically, such as those containing anabolic agents or steroids, should be avoided. These can have serious side effects, particularly for older adults, and some are banned from sports and other activities. Additionally, be cautious with weight loss pills or energy boosters that contain large amounts of caffeine or other stimulants. While they might offer a temporary energy spike, they can lead to heart palpitations, high blood pressure, and sleep disturbances, which are particularly risky for seniors.

The dietary supplement industry is not regulated like prescription medications are, which means there is considerable variability in the quality and purity of products available. To ensure a safe and effective product, look for supplements certified by third-party organizations such as the U.S. Pharmacopeia (USP), NSF International, or ConsumerLab.com. These companies test supplements to verify that they contain the ingredients listed on the label and are free from harmful contaminants.

Before adding any supplement to your routine, consult with healthcare providers, especially if you have pre-existing health conditions or are taking medications. Interactions between supplements and medications can occur, and what is safe for one person may not be for another. For instance, omega-3 supplements can thin the blood, which can be dangerous if you're taking blood-thinning medications. A healthcare provider can help you assess whether a particular supplement is necessary and safe for you and can help you determine the correct dosage to meet your individual needs.

By approaching supplements with informed caution and professional guidance, you can safely incorporate those that may benefit your health and support your strength training efforts. Remember, supplements should not replace a balanced diet but be used to fill nutritional gaps. With the right strategy, you can enhance muscle recovery, support overall health, and thrive in your fitness endeavors.

4.4 Understanding and Managing Post-workout Soreness

After a fulfilling session of strength training, feeling some muscle soreness is common, especially if you're either new to exercise or have recently intensified your workout. This phenomenon, often known as delayed onset muscle soreness (DOMS), occurs due to micro-tears in the muscle fibers caused by exertion. Essentially, when you engage in physical activities that are new to your body or when you push your muscles harder than usual, it results in tiny tears. These tears are a natural and necessary part of building stronger muscles; as these tears repair, your muscles grow more robust. However, the accompanying soreness can range from mildly uncomfortable to painful, making your next workout daunting.

Managing this soreness can help you stay on track with your training program without discomfort. One of the most accessible and natural methods to alleviate muscle soreness is applying cold and heat therapies. Cold therapy (ice packs) can be particularly effective immediately after your workout and for up to 48 hours afterward. The cold helps reduce inflammation and numbs the sore areas, providing quick relief. On the other hand, heat therapy, which can be a warm bath or a heating pad, is excellent for relaxing and loosening stiff muscles and improving blood flow, which aids in the recovery process. This increase in circulation helps flush out the metabolic waste products accumulated in the muscles during exercise.

Gentle stretching and massage are other effective strategies for managing post-workout soreness. Light stretching after a workout can help reduce muscle tension and increase flexibility, thus easing the discomfort of DOMS. Similarly, massage can significantly alleviate muscle tightness and soreness, whether self-administered or performed by a professional. It improves muscle circulation, which, like heat therapy, helps remove toxins and brings nutrients that aid recovery. Using foam rollers or massage balls to perform self-myofascial release can also be particularly effective in targeting specific sore spots. Easily incorporate it into your cool-down routine.

While muscle soreness is a normal response to exertion, understanding when this soreness might indicate a potential injury is crucial. Normal muscle soreness peaks within 24 to 72 hours after exercise and gradually subsides. Soreness is often described as a dull, aching pain accompanying muscle stiffness. However, if you experience sharp, intense, or persistent pain that doesn't improve with rest and natural remedies, it could be a sign of injury, such as a muscle strain or tear. Additionally, if you have significant swelling, redness, or warmth, these could be signs of more severe conditions like inflammation or infection, and you should seek medical attention.

When experiencing excessive soreness, it's essential to adjust your workouts accordingly. Active recovery can be beneficial—but you may need to modify the intensity and volume of your exercises. For instance, if your legs are particularly sore from squatting, consider focusing on upper body exercises in your next session or engage in low-impact activities such as walking or swimming, which can help maintain mobility and circulation without exacerbating the soreness. Listening to your body and scaling back when necessary is not a setback but a way to ensure longevity in your training regimen.

4.5 Sleep's Role in Muscle Recovery

The rejuvenating power of sleep extends far beyond just erasing the signs of a tiring day; it's a fundamental pillar in the recovery process, particularly when you engage in strength training. During sleep, your body goes into overdrive, repairing muscle fibers damaged during workouts. This process matters because it's not the act of lifting weights that builds muscle but rather the recovery afterward when the tissues heal and grow stronger. Growth hormone, which plays an essential role in tissue growth and muscle repair, is primarily released during deep sleep. Getting adequate rest is not a luxury but necessary for anyone looking to improve their strength and overall fitness.

Improving the quality of your sleep can significantly enhance these recovery processes. Establishing a consistent bedtime routine is one of the most effective strategies. A routine might include activities that help signal to your body that it's time to wind down, such as reading a book, taking a warm bath, or practicing gentle yoga or meditation. These activities help ease the transition into sleep, making it quicker and more restful. Consider temperature, noise levels, and lighting to optimize your bedroom for comfort and relaxation. Ensuring your mattress and pillows provide the appropriate support and comfort can also make a substantial difference in sleep quality. These adjustments might seem small, but they can significantly impact how quickly you fall asleep and how deeply you sleep, facilitating better muscle recovery.

Understanding your changing sleep needs as you age is vital. Older adults often experience changes in sleep patterns, including increased wakefulness during the night and earlier waking times, which can interfere with the deep sleep needed for adequate muscle recovery. Adjust your sleep schedule by aiming for earlier bedtimes and daily naps to compensate for deficits. Please pay attention to your diet and exercise related to sleep; avoiding caffeine late in the day and engaging in regular physical activity can promote better sleep. Exercising too close to bedtime can be stimulating, whereas finishing workouts a few hours before can help enhance sleep quality.

Numerous studies support the link between sleep and strength training performance. Better sleep improves muscle recovery, higher energy levels, and better workout performance. When well-rested, your mind and body are better prepared to handle the physical demands of strength training. You can focus better, maintain better form, and have the energy to complete your workout effectively.

On the other hand, insufficient sleep can lead to decreased performance, slower reaction times, and a higher risk of injuries.

4.6 Active Recovery Techniques

Active recovery is a gentle yet powerful tool that complements strength training efforts. Unlike passive recovery, which involves complete rest, active recovery involves engaging in low-intensity exercise that stimulates muscle recovery without imposing undue strain. The beauty of active recovery lies in its dual ability to enhance muscle repair and mitigate stiffness, making it particularly beneficial as we age.

Active recovery helps maintain blood flow to the muscles, which can help flush out metabolic waste products accumulated during intense physical activity. Enhanced blood circulation not only speeds up tissue repair but also reduces muscle stiffness and soreness. Walking, gentle yoga, and light swimming are perfect examples of active recovery exercises. These activities keep the body moving and engaged without the intensity of regular training sessions, providing a balance that helps maintain physical fitness while allowing the body to recover.

Tips for Effective Stretching:

- **Breathe Deeply**: Inhale and exhale slowly during each stretch.
- **Avoid Bouncing**: Hold each stretch steadily without bouncing to prevent injury.
- **Listen to Your Body**: Stretch to mild discomfort but not pain.

Monitoring your recovery is essential to ensure you're giving your body what it needs to repair and strengthen. Pay attention to how your body feels on the days following different types of workouts and recovery activities. Signs of adequate recovery include decreased muscle soreness, feeling energized rather than tired, and a readiness to perform at your usual level during your next workout session. If you feel unusually tired, experiencing persistent soreness, or unable to perform at your typical level, it may be a sign that you need to allow more time for recovery or adjust the intensity of your active recovery activities.

A good post-workout stretching routine should focus on flexibility, mobility, and relaxation. Here is a simple and effective exercise that targets major muscle groups and can be done in about 10-15 minutes:

Hamstring Stretch

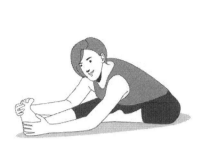 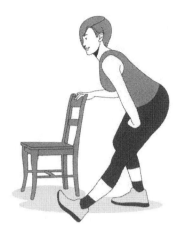

- **How to do it**: Sit on the floor with one leg extended and the other bent so that the sole is against the inner thigh of the extended leg. Reach for the toes of the extended leg. You can also do this while standing with support.
- **Hold** 20-30 seconds for each leg.
- **Benefits**: Stretches the hamstrings and lower back.

Quadriceps Stretch

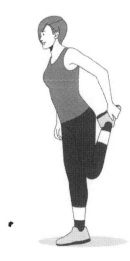

- **How to do it**: Stand on one leg and pull the opposite foot toward the buttocks, keeping the knees close together.
- **Hold** 20-30 seconds for each leg.
- **Benefits**: Stretches the front of the thigh.

Calf Stretch

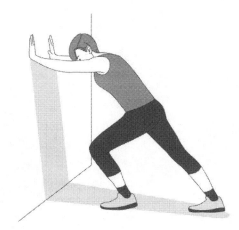

- **How to do it**: Stand facing a wall. Place hands on the wall at shoulder height, step one foot back, keep the foot flat on the floor, bend the front knee, and lean forward.
- **Hold** 20-30 seconds for each leg.
- **Benefits**: Stretches the calf muscles.

Hip Flexor Stretch

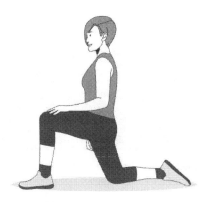

- **How to do it**: Kneel on one knee with the other foot in front, creating a 90-degree angle at both knees. Gently push the hips forward.
- **Hold** 20-30 seconds for each side.
- **Benefits**: Stretches the hip flexors and quads.

Shoulder Stretch

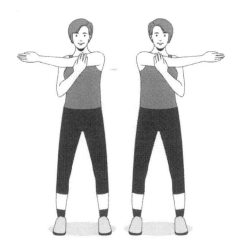

- **How to do it**: Bring one arm across the body and use the opposite arm to pull it closer to the chest gently.
- **Hold** 20-30 seconds for each arm.
- **Benefits**: Stretches the shoulders and upper back.

Chest Stretch

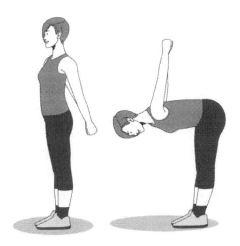

A chest stretch, completed by clasping hands behind your back, is an effective way to open up the chest and shoulders, improving flexibility and posture. You can also make this easier by grasping a towel in each hand, easing the pull on the chest until you are more flexible.

Lower Back Stretch

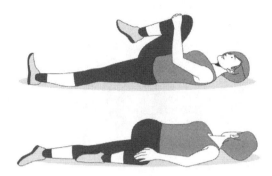

- **How to do it**: Lie on your back, hug your knees to your chest, and gently rock side to side. Then, hug one knee in at a time. Cross your knee over and get a spinal twist if it is comfortable.
- **Hold**: 20-30 seconds.
- **Benefits**: Stretches the lower back and relieves tension.

4.7 Menopausal Weight Gain and Nutritional Needs

"Women's metabolisms slow about 10 years earlier than they do for men. Gaining weight isn't a given. You just have to be that much more diligent about exercise and what you eat due to that metabolic difference."

- Mary Weiler, nutrition scientist at Abbott specializing in women's health

Belly Fat in Menopausal Women

Menopausal weight gain affects about 60-70% of women going through menopause. This weight gain is often due to a decrease in muscle mass caused by hormonal changes. These hormone shifts also cause more fat to gather around the belly. One study found that women in the perimenopausal stage doubled their fat mass before menopause. Belly fat can lead to health problems, such as insulin resistance, higher risks of certain cancers, and heart issues like high blood pressure, obesity, and abnormal cholesterol levels.

Hormonal Shifts Related to Menopause

In the United States, the average age for menopause is usually between 47 and 55. As women approach midlife, they will notice hormonal changes like irregular periods, which eventually stop. During menopause, the ovaries stop producing hormones. Menopause symptoms happen due to changing hormones and usually decrease after menopause, but risks like heart disease and bone loss may continue. The table below shows the common hormones that change during menopause and their effects on weight gain. You can ask your doctor to test your hormone levels, and online labs will send you a home kit.

Hormone	Description	Effects of Decrease on Weight Gain
Estrogen	This primary female sex hormone regulates the menstrual cycle, reproductive system, and secondary sexual characteristics.	• Increased abdominal fat • Redistribution of body fat • Decreased muscle mass, leading to a slower metabolism
Progesterone	This hormone prepares the uterus for pregnancy and maintains the early stages of pregnancy. It works with estrogen to regulate the menstrual cycle.	• Water retention and bloating • Increased appetite and cravings
Testosterone	This hormone is responsible for libido, muscle mass, and energy levels. It is present in lower amounts in women compared to men.	• Decreased muscle mass, leading to a slower metabolism • Increased body fat, particularly abdominal fat
DHEA (Dehydroepiandrosterone)	This is a precursor hormone that converts into estrogen and testosterone. It is essential for overall hormonal balance and wellbeing.	• Increased body fat, particularly abdominal fat
Thyroid Hormones (T3 and T4)	These hormones regulate metabolism, energy production, and overall metabolic rate.	• Slowed metabolism • Weight gain • Difficulty losing weight
Cortisol	This stress hormone is produced by the adrenal glands. It regulates metabolism, immune response, and stress response.	• Chronic elevated cortisol levels lead to increased abdominal fat • Increased appetite and cravings for high-calorie foods • Insulin resistance and weight gain

1. Estrogen

- **Test**: Blood test or saliva test
- **Purpose**: Measures the level of estrogen, which is essential for reproductive health, bone density, and regulating the menstrual cycle.
- **Preparation**: Check to see if there is a specific time to take this test.

2. Progesterone

- **Test**: Blood test or saliva test
- **Purpose**: Measures the level of progesterone, which is crucial for regulating the menstrual cycle and maintaining pregnancy.
- **Preparation**: For women, testing is usually done during the luteal phase of the menstrual cycle, typically about 7 days after ovulation.

3. Testosterone

- **Test**: Blood test or saliva test
- **Purpose**: Measures the level of testosterone, which is important for reproductive health, muscle mass, and overall vitality in both men and women.
- **Preparation**: Testosterone levels can fluctuate throughout the day, so tests are often done in the morning when levels are typically highest.

5. DHEA (Dehydroepiandrosterone)

- **Test**: Blood test or saliva test
- **Purpose**: Measures the level of DHEA, a hormone involved in producing other hormones like estrogen and testosterone.
- **Preparation**: No special preparation is usually needed, but follow your doctor's instructions if any specific guidelines are given.

5. Thyroid Hormones (T3 and T4)

- **Test**: Blood test
  - T3 (Triiodothyronine): Measures the level of T3, which regulates metabolism.
  - T4 (Thyroxine): Measures the level of T4, the primary hormone produced by the thyroid gland.
- **Purpose**: Evaluate thyroid function, which affects metabolism, energy levels, and overall hormonal balance.
- **Preparation**: No special preparation is usually needed.

6. Cortisol

- **Test**: Blood test, urine test, or saliva test
- **Purpose**: Measures the level of cortisol, a hormone produced by the adrenal glands in response to stress and involved in regulating metabolism, immune response, and circadian rhythms.
- **Preparation**: Cortisol levels vary throughout the day, so tests are often conducted in the morning when levels are highest, or multiple samples may be taken throughout the day to assess the daily pattern.

The 5-Step Approach to Reducing Belly Fat and Improving Health

Eliminating menopausal belly fat can be challenging due to hormonal changes, but focusing on a balanced diet can help manage and reduce it. Here are some foods that can be particularly beneficial:

→ Step 1: Eat as Clean as You Can

Lean Proteins–Examples: Chicken breast, turkey, fish, tofu, beans. Helps maintain muscle mass, which can boost metabolism.

High-Fiber Foods–Examples: Vegetables (broccoli, spinach), fruits (berries, apples), whole grains (oats, quinoa), legumes (lentils, chickpeas). Promotes fullness, regulates blood sugar, and improves digestive health.

Healthy Fats–Examples: Avocados, nuts, seeds, olive oil, fatty fish (salmon, mackerel). Supports heart health and hormone balance and can help reduce inflammation.

Low-Glycemic Index Foods–Examples: Whole grains, sweet potatoes, non-starchy vegetables. Stabilizes blood sugar levels, which can help prevent insulin spikes that contribute to fat storage.

Fermented Foods–Examples: Yogurt, kefir, sauerkraut, kimchi. Improves gut health, impacting overall weight management and reducing bloating.

Green Tea–Benefits: Contains antioxidants like catechins that may boost metabolism and aid in fat loss.

Water-Rich Foods–Examples: Cucumbers, watermelon, celery. Helps keep you hydrated and may reduce bloating.

→ Step 2: Portion Control: Being Mindful of Portion Sizes Can Help Manage Calorie Intake

Example: Caloric Intake for a Lightly Active 50-Year-Old Woman is ~1800

Lightly Active: Include activity or moderate activity about two to three times a week. There are several calorie calculators, such as this one from the Mayo Clinic:

https://www.mayoclinic.org/healthy-lifestyle/weight-loss/in-depth/calorie-calculator/itt-20402304

This calorie count is just an estimate that you should take into consideration when eating. If you are logging your meals in your journal and adding up the calories and find that you are eating 2500 calories a day, then you now have information that you can take action on—reducing your caloric intake to lose weight. You can also calculate your Basal Metabolic Rate which is the number of calories you should have if you didn't do anything active in 24 hours. This will give you another data point in order to make some informed decisions. I don't recommend calorie counting as a long-term tool, because it is onerous and boring, but as a start for the first week or so of your journey, it is absolutely beneficial.

https://www.myfitnesspal.com/tools/bmr-calculator

→ Step 3: Limit Certain Foods and Practice Mindful Eating

Reducing your intake of processed foods high in sugar and unhealthy fats can prevent excess calorie consumption and weight gain. These foods include candy, potato chips, fried foods, soda, energy drinks, and baked goods. Limit your alcohol intake.

Mindful eating involves slowing down and focusing on our eating habits, helping us recognize if we are full sooner, thus preventing overeating and weight gain. It requires time and effort.

Tips include:
- Eating slowly so you can stop when you are 80% full.
- Dedicating mealtimes without distractions.
- Planning meals intentionally.

→ **Step 4: Manage Stress**

High stress can lead to weight gain, so practices like yoga, meditation, or deep breathing can be beneficial.

→ **Step 5: Sleep Quality**

Poor sleep is linked to weight gain, so ensuring adequate, quality sleep is important.

- **Stick to a Sleep Schedule:** Go to bed and wake up at the same time every day to regulate your sleep cycle.
- **Avoid Late Naps**: Try not to nap in the late afternoon or evening to prevent difficulty falling asleep at night.
- **Create a Bedtime Routine:** Develop relaxing activities before bed like reading, listening to calming music, or taking a warm bath.
- **Limit Screen Time:** Avoid watching TV or using computers and phones in the bedroom, as the light can interfere with your ability to fall asleep.
- **Maintain a Comfortable Bedroom Environment:** Keep your bedroom cool, quiet, and comfortable to promote better sleep.
- **Exercise Regularly:** Exercise daily, but avoid working out close to bedtime.
- **Watch Your Diet:** Avoid large meals close to bedtime and limit caffeine intake from coffee, tea, and chocolate late in the day.
- **Limit Alcohol:** Avoid alcohol before bed, as even small amounts can disrupt your sleep.

Choose Foods that Take Longer to Digest

Studies show that a low-glycemic index (GI) diet can help manage weight and blood sugar levels during menopause. The glycemic index measures how much a food raises blood sugar and insulin levels. While no single food can target belly fat specifically, combining these foods as part of a balanced diet and healthy lifestyle can contribute to overall weight management and reduction of menopausal belly fat

- High-GI foods (score of 70 or higher) are digested quickly.
- Moderate-GI foods (score of 56-69) have a moderate impact.
- Low-GI foods (score of less than 55) are digested slowly.

To get started, focus on a low-GI Mediterranean diet. This diet includes:

- Lean meats, fatty fish, and poultry
- Healthy fats such as nuts, seeds, avocados, and extra virgin olive oil
- Moderate amounts of beans, lentils, and whole grains
- Plenty of low-GI fruits and vegetables, such as apples, pears, berries, oranges, leafy greens, cruciferous vegetables, carrots, tomatoes, cucumbers, celery, and green beans

Overnight chocolate chia seed pudding is a delicious snack, especially if you have the "munchies" or a sweet tooth.

Here's my recipe:

Blend 2 cups of milk (see chart to choose), 0.5 cups of chia seeds (if you don't like the crunch, you can put these in a coffee grinder first), 0.25 cups of unsweetened dark cocoa powder, 2 Tablespoons of honey, 1 teaspoon of vanilla extract, and 0.5 teaspoons of cinnamon.

Nutrient	Plant-Based Milk (Per Serving)	Cow's Milk 2% (Per Serving)
Calories	180.4	221.4
Protein	10.7 grams	15.2 grams
Fat	9.1 grams	10.2 grams
Carbs	17.1 grams	21.1 grams
Fiber	5.9 grams	5.9 grams
Sugar	9.9 grams	15.4 grams

Benefits of Chia Seeds

Chia seeds are a nutrient-dense food with numerous health benefits:

1. **High in Nutrients**: Chia seeds are rich in fiber, protein, omega-3 fatty acids, antioxidants, and various micronutrients such as calcium, magnesium, and phosphorus.
2. **Rich in Antioxidants**: They contain antioxidants that help protect the body from free radicals, aging, and cancer.
3. **Excellent Source of Fiber**: The high fiber content aids digestion, helps maintain healthy bowel movements, and can contribute to weight management by promoting a feeling of fullness.
4. **Omega-3 Fatty Acids**: Chia seeds are one of the best plant-based sources of omega-3 fatty acids, which benefit heart health.
5. **Supports Bone Health**: They are high in calcium, magnesium, and phosphorus, essential for maintaining strong bones.
6. **Blood Sugar Regulation**: Chia seeds' fiber and protein content can help regulate blood sugar levels, which is beneficial for managing diabetes.
7. **Heart Health**: Chia seeds can help improve cholesterol levels, reducing the risk of heart disease.
8. **Weight Management**: Chia seeds' high fiber content can help promote satiety and reduce overall calorie intake.
9. **Hydration**: When soaked in water, chia seeds can absorb up to 12 times their weight in liquid, which can help keep the body hydrated.

Incorporating chia seeds into your diet, such as in this pudding recipe, can provide numerous health benefits and contribute to overall well-being.

As we wrap up this chapter, it's clear that the synergy between proper nutrition, hydration, smart supplementation, and thoughtful recovery practices forms the backbone of a successful strength training regimen. Each element helps you achieve and maintain your fitness goals, ensuring you can continue leading an active and vibrant life.

Make a Difference with Your Review

Unlock the Power of Generosity

"The greatest gift you can give someone is the strength to stand tall."

- Jessie Hilgenberg, an IFBB Figure Pro

As women, we know that true strength comes not just from muscles but from the heart. It's about lifting each other up, sharing our wisdom, and helping one another grow stronger in every way.

With that in mind, I have a simple question for you...

Would you help someone you've never met, even if no one knew it was you?

That person could be someone just like you—or like you were before you discovered the benefits of strength training. She might feel unsure and overwhelmed and need guidance to start her journey to better health and confidence.

Our mission at Sage Lifestyle Press is to make strength training accessible and encouraging for every woman, especially those in midlife and beyond. But we can't do it alone. To reach as many women as possible, we need your help.

This is where you come in. People judge a book by its reviews, and your words could encourage another woman to start gaining the confidence that comes from strength training today.

So here's my heartfelt request on behalf of a woman you've never met:

Please take a moment to leave a review for *Beginner's Guide to Strength Training for Women Over 50*.

Your kind words cost nothing but can mean everything to someone else. Your review could help...

- One more woman finds the strength to start.
- One more woman realizes it's never too late.
- One more woman feels confident in her body again.
- One more woman reclaims her vitality.

To make a difference, all it takes is 60 seconds of your time. Simply scan the QR code below to leave your review:

If helping another woman find her strength makes you smile, you're already one of us. Welcome to the club.

Thank you for joining us on this journey. We're excited to see how strong you'll become and to help you achieve your goals even faster and easier with the strategies shared in this book.

With gratitude,

Sage Lifestyle Press

P.S. - When you share something valuable, you become valuable too. If you think this book could help another woman in your life, don't hesitate to share it with her.

5

Next Steps—Building Your Own Routines

As we embrace the world of strength training, creating a structured and well-thought-out weekly plan is like drawing a map for a treasure hunt. It guides you through each step of your fitness adventure, ensuring that every workout brings you closer to your goals while keeping health and safety at the forefront. Just as a seasoned captain navigates a ship through both calm and stormy waters, we must learn to balance and adjust our fitness routines to suit our body's needs and life's unpredictability.

5.1 Designing Your Weekly Strength Training Plan

Balancing Frequency and Intensity

The secret to a successful strength training program, especially for those of us in midlife, is finding the perfect balance between how often (frequency) and how hard (intensity) we train. It's about stimulating muscle growth and improvements without overburdening our bodies, thus minimizing the risk of injury. A balanced plan involves varying the intensity of your workouts; some days might be more challenging, pushing you to your limits, while others might be easier, allowing your body to recover. For instance, after a day of focusing on heavier weights, you might follow up with a session that uses lighter weights, or even body resistance. This variation keeps your muscles guessing, which is excellent for continued improvement and reduces the risk of strain from overuse.

When planning the frequency of your workouts, consider starting with two to three sessions per week. This schedule allows ample muscle recovery downtime, which is crucial for growth and strength enhancement. You may increase this frequency as you grow more robust and comfortable, but always listen to your body's cues. Overtraining can lead to fatigue and soreness, counteracting the benefits of your hard work.

Adapting Plans to Energy Levels

Our energy levels can fluctuate based on numerous factors—everything from sleep quality to daily stress can play a role. Therefore, it is important to be flexible and willing to adjust your workout plan according to how you feel each day. If you wake up feeling energetic and strong, you might choose to tackle a more challenging workout. Conversely, a lighter workout—or even additional rest—might be more beneficial on days you feel drained.

This adaptable approach ensures that you are working with your body, not against it, promoting long-term health and fitness. The important thing is to make strength training a priority in your weekly regimen. This strategy not only helps you achieve your fitness goals but also enhances your overall wellbeing, allowing you to enjoy the myriad benefits of an active lifestyle. As you continue to apply these principles, your ability to handle the physical demands of strength training improves, along with your overall energy and vitality.

5.2 Integrating Strength Training with Other Types of Exercise

Introducing a variety of exercises into your weekly routine is not just about keeping boredom at bay—it's a strategic approach to enhancing your overall fitness and preventing injuries. While strength training forms the core of building muscle and increasing bone density, incorporating cardiovascular exercises into your regimen can significantly boost your heart health and endurance.

Cardiovascular activities, such as brisk walking or swimming, elevate your heart rate, which helps to improve heart and lung function while burning calories. When integrating cardio with strength training, consider alternating days between these activities. For instance, if you engage in strength training on Monday, Wednesday, and Friday, schedule your cardiovascular workouts for Tuesday and Thursday. This alternating schedule allows you to work out different muscle groups and systems without overloading, reducing the risk of injury and fatigue.

Flexibility and balance exercises like yoga or Tai Chi are a great addition to a well-rounded fitness plan. These practices enhance your range of motion, help prevent falls by improving your balance, support muscle recovery, and reduce stress. Incorporating these activities once or twice a week can complement your strength training and cardio routines by allowing your muscles to heal and realign. For example, a gentle yoga session after a strength training day can help elongate the muscles worked, aiding in recovery and reducing stiffness. Tai Chi, often called "meditation in motion," can be especially beneficial for those looking for a low-impact option emphasizing slow, controlled movements to enhance balance and mental focus.

Variety in your activities is key to a sustainable exercise habit. To keep things interesting, try new classes or activities every few months. This could mean joining a dance class, trying out a new fitness class at your local community center, or even taking up a sport like golf or pickleball. These activities introduce you to different forms of exercise and provide social opportunities, which can be incredibly enriching. The social aspect of trying out new classes or sports can also be motivating, making you more likely to stick with your fitness goals. Additionally, consider seasonal variations in your activities; for example, if you enjoy outdoor activities, you might switch to indoor cycling or aqua aerobics during the colder months. This keeps your routine adaptable to weather conditions and introduces you to different exercise formats that can work for other muscle groups or challenge you in new ways.

By integrating a mix of strength training, cardiovascular exercises, flexibility, and balance activities and engaging in cross-training, you create a dynamic and responsive fitness regimen that caters to all aspects of your physical health. This approach enhances your overall fitness and well-being and keeps your exercise routine enjoyable and exciting. As you continue to explore and integrate these various forms of exercise into your life, remember that each has unique benefits that contribute to a healthier, more vibrant you. Embrace the diversity of exercise options available, and enjoy the journey toward a fitter, happier self.

5.3 Setting Realistic Goals and Milestones

SMART Goals

When embarking on your fitness journey, it's crucial to set goals that challenge you and are realistically achievable. This is where SMART goals come into the picture. SMART stands for Specific, Measurable, Achievable, Relevant, and Time-bound. Each element of this acronym guides you in setting well-defined and trackable goals, increasing the likelihood of success. For instance, a SMART goal around strength training could be, "I will do three strength training sessions each week for the next month to increase my upper body strength." This goal is specific (attending strength training sessions), measurable (three sessions each week), achievable (a realistic number of sessions in a week), relevant (improves a desired area of fitness), and time-bound (set for the next month).

When applying SMART goals to your fitness planning, clearly define your goal. Consider why each goal is important to you to help keep your motivation high. Then, consider how you can measure your progress toward this goal. It could be tracking the number of workouts, monitoring the weights you lift, or noting how your body feels and performs. Making your goals achievable is about understanding your current fitness level and setting a goal that is a stretch, yet within reach. Ensure your goals are relevant to your overall fitness aspirations, and finally, give yourself a deadline to aim for, which creates a sense of urgency and helps maintain your focus.

Setting Short-term and Long-term Goals

Having a mix of short-term and long-term goals is helpful for sustaining motivation throughout your fitness journey. Short-term goals serve as stepping-stones to more significant achievements and provide frequent moments of accomplishment that boost your morale. For example, a short-term goal might be to learn the proper form for five new strength training exercises within two weeks. On the other hand, long-term goals focus on bigger achievements that require persistent effort.

Balancing these goals allows you to celebrate immediate successes while keeping your eyes on the broader prize, helping to maintain a positive and proactive mindset. It's like crafting a tapestry, where each small stitch contributes to creating a beautiful and complete picture. Regularly achieving short-term goals builds confidence and compounds your progress toward more ambitious, long-term goals. Keeping your fitness journal will make reviewing and seeing your achievements easy.

Adjusting Goals Based on Progress

As you progress in your strength training, your abilities and circumstances might change, which means your goals may also need to evolve. Periodically assessing your progress is critical. If you exceed your targets, it might be time to set more challenging ones. Conversely, if a goal seems too difficult to achieve, consider breaking it down into smaller, more manageable pieces or extending your timeframe.

This flexible approach ensures that your goals remain appropriate for your current fitness level and life circumstances, keeping you well-rested and calm. It's about finding that sweet spot where each goal pushes you just enough to continue making meaningful progress.

Celebrating Milestones

Remember, every achievement, big or small, deserves recognition. Celebrating milestones acknowledges your hard work and dedication and reinforces your commitment to your fitness journey. Whether treating yourself to a new workout outfit after reaching a particular strength milestone or simply reflecting on your progress with a friend, recognizing how far you've come is crucial.

By integrating these strategies—setting SMART goals, balancing short-term and long-term objectives, adjusting goals as needed, and celebrating milestones—you create a dynamic and responsive approach to fitness that adapts to your evolving needs and achievements. This method maximizes your potential in achieving and surpassing your fitness goals and ensures the journey is enjoyable and rewarding. As you continue navigating your fitness plan, remember that each goal, each adjustment, and each celebration brings you one step closer to realizing your health and wellness aspirations.

5.4 When to Upscale Your Exercises

As you continue to engage in regular strength training, there comes a time when your current routine may start to feel more comfortable, and the once-challenging weights might not make you exert as much effort as before. This is a natural part of fitness progression and a sign that your body is adapting and getting stronger. Recognizing the right moment to increase the intensity or complexity of your workouts is crucial to continue making gains and improving your fitness level.

One of the primary indicators that you are ready to take your workouts up a notch is the ease with which you complete your current exercises. If you can perform your sets without much exertion, or if the last few repetitions no longer challenge you, it's likely time to increase the intensity. Additionally, suppose your recovery time between sessions has significantly decreased, and you feel less tired after workouts. This also signals that your body has adapted to the current demands, making it the perfect time to introduce more challenging elements into your routine.

Increasing the intensity of your workouts can be achieved in several ways. One straightforward method is to add more weight to your exercises. Gradually increasing your weight stimulates muscle growth and enhances bone density, which is particularly beneficial as we age. Another method is to increase the number of repetitions or sets you perform. This approach, often called volume training, can help improve endurance and muscle tone.

However, keeping safety at the forefront is essential to upscaling your exercises. Ensure that any increase in weight or intensity is gradual to avoid overloading your muscles and joints. Maintaining proper form throughout each exercise is crucial to prevent injuries. Pay close attention to your body's responses to the increased demands. Mild soreness after a workout is typical, but sharp pain or discomfort that lasts more than a few days is a sign that you may be pushing too hard.

Upscaling your exercises is a natural progression in your strength training journey. By recognizing the signs of readiness, understanding how to increase workout intensity safely, and seeking professional guidance, you can ensure that your fitness regimen continues challenging you, promoting further improvements in strength, endurance, and overall health. As you implement these changes, remember to listen to your body and adjust your routines as needed, allowing you to enjoy the benefits of an active lifestyle safely and enjoyably.

As we conclude this chapter on building effective and personalized routines, remember that tracking and adjusting are continuous. Each data, recorded entry, and reflected feeling contribute to a deeper understanding of your body and its needs, guiding you toward more tailored and effective workouts. This meticulous approach to tracking and adjusting ensures that your fitness regimen remains dynamic, responsive, and, most importantly, aligned with your evolving health goals and lifestyle needs.

The next chapter will explore advanced techniques and strategies to enhance your training regimen further. From exploring new exercise modalities to understanding how to integrate them effectively into your routine, we will delve deeper into making your fitness journey effective and genuinely transformative.

6

Advanced Techniques and Strategies

As you evolve in your strength training journey, embracing advanced techniques and strategies can significantly enhance your results, keeping your routine both challenging and exciting. Think of these advanced methods as your fitness spice rack—just as the right combination of spices can transform a meal, integrating new exercises and tools can revitalize your workouts, providing fresh challenges and renewed motivation.

6.1 Incorporating Resistance Bands into Your Routine

Resistance bands, those stretchy strips of rubber that can vary in thickness and length, are a powerhouse tool for enhancing your workout regimen. Their unique benefits stem from the continuous tension they provide. Unlike free weights, where the tension decreases as you complete the motion, resistance bands maintain a consistent load, challenging your muscles from the start of the exercise to its completion. This constant tension improves coordination and increases the stabilization demands on your body, boosting joint stability and strengthening muscles at various angles—capabilities that are particularly beneficial as we age.

Integrating resistance bands with free weights can elevate the intensity of your workouts without putting undue stress on your joints. This combination allows you to engage more muscle groups simultaneously, enhancing the efficiency of your workouts. For instance, consider a bicep curl with a resistance band and a dumbbell. As you curl the dumbbell, the resistance band intensifies the challenge, especially at the point of the exercise where the dumbbell becomes more accessible to lift, ensuring your muscles work hard throughout the entire movement. This method increases muscle strength, promotes muscle endurance, and speeds up metabolic rates, which can be a boon for weight management.

Let's explore a variety of exercises that utilize resistance bands to target both the upper and lower body, ensuring a comprehensive workout. For the upper body, try the resistance band pull-apart. Hold a resistance band with both hands in front of you at chest level, then pull the band apart while keeping your arms straight, engaging the muscles in your shoulders and upper back. For the lower body, the resistance band squat adds a delightful challenge. Place a resistance band around your thighs just above your knees, and as you squat, the band adds extra resistance, making your muscles work harder to maintain proper form and posture.

Safety is paramount when using resistance bands. Always inspect your bands before use for any signs of wear and tear, such as small tears or thinning, which could lead to the band snapping during exercise—a potential injury risk. Start with a lighter resistance band and gradually work toward higher resistances to build your strength safely. Ensure the band is securely anchored under your feet or to a sturdy object to prevent it from slipping and causing injury. Additionally, when performing exercises, ensure that you control the movements of exertion and release to keep the band stable and effective.

By incorporating resistance bands into your strength training routine, you not only diversify your workouts but also introduce a flexible, effective tool that enhances muscle strength, coordination, and overall fitness. Whether used alone or combined with free weights, resistance bands can provide a low-cost, high-impact method of ensuring your workouts remain robust, varied, and tailored to your advancing fitness needs. As you integrate these versatile tools into your routine, embrace the challenge they bring and enjoy the tangible benefits they deliver to your strength training practice.

6.2 Advanced Workout Options

In the fitness landscape, especially as we navigate our 50s and beyond, cultivating balance isn't just about achieving a physical equilibrium; it's about laying the groundwork for sustained mobility and independence. Balance training's critical role becomes increasingly important as it directly contributes to reducing the risk of falls—a common concern for many of us in this age group. More-over, well-honed balance enhances overall mobility, making everyday activities smoother and safer.

One of the most effective ways to elevate your balance training is by incorporating dynamic balance exercises that challenge your body in new and varied ways. Exercises like deadlifts provide a fantastic way to engage and strengthen the muscles that stabilize your hips, knees, and ankles. The deadlift targets the hamstrings, glutes, lower back, and core muscles, improving balance and stability.

Deadlifts

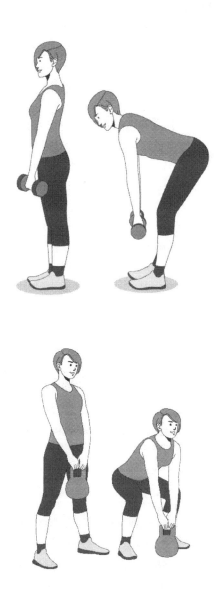

Setup:

- Choose two comfortable-weight dumbbells or a kettlebell. Beginners should start with lighter weights to ensure proper form.

Starting Position:

- Stand with your feet shoulder-width apart.
- Use an overhand grip with palm(s) facing your body.
- Keep your back straight, chest up, and shoulders back. Your knees should be slightly bent, not locked.

Execution:

- Hinge at your hips, pushing them back as you lower toward the ground.
- Keep the weight(s) close to your legs, maintaining a straight back throughout the movement.
- Lower the weight(s) until they are at mid-shin level or just above the ground, depending on your flexibility.
- Drive through your heels to push your hips forward, lifting the weight(s) back up.
- Keep your back straight and engage your glutes as you return to the starting position.
- Stand tall at the top of the movement, ensuring your shoulders are back and your chest is up.

Breathing:

- Take a deep breath as you lower the dumbbells.
- Breathe out as you lift the dumbbells back to the starting position.

Tips for Proper Form:

- **Keep the Core Engaged**: Maintain tension in your core throughout the exercise to protect your lower back.
- **Avoid Rounding the Back**: Keep your back straight to prevent injury.
- **Control the Movement**: Perform the exercise in a controlled manner, avoiding any jerky movements.
- **Focus on the Hips**: The movement should be driven by your hips rather than your lower back or knees.

Common Mistakes to Avoid:

- **Using Too Much Weight**: Start with a manageable weight to master the form before increasing the load.
- **Locking Knees**: Keep slightly bending your knees to avoid straining them.
- **Rounding the Back**: Ensure your back remains straight to prevent injury.
- **Hyperextending the Back**: Do not arch your back at the top of the movement; keep it neutral.

Sumo Squats

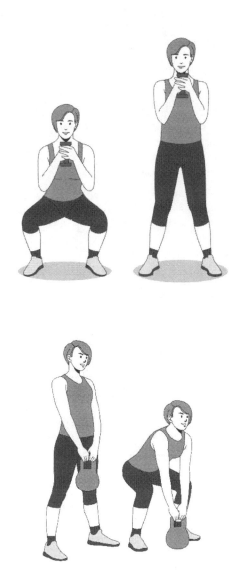

The sumo squat is a variation of the traditional squat that targets the inner thighs, glutes, and quads. It's an excellent exercise for building lower body strength and improving flexibility. Here's how to perform the sumo squat:

Setup:

- Stand with your feet wider than shoulder-width apart, toes pointing out at a 45-degree angle.
- Keep your chest up, shoulders back, and core engaged.
- If you aren't using weight, then place your hands on your hips, hold them before you, or clasp them at your chest for balance.

Execution:

Squat Down:
- Lower your body by bending at your hips and knees, keeping your back straight and chest lifted.
- Push your knees outward, in line with your toes, as you descend. This helps to engage your inner thighs.
- Aim to lower yourself until your thighs are parallel to the ground or as low as you can comfortably go while maintaining proper form.

Pause:
- Hold the squat position for a moment at the bottom, feeling the stretch in your inner thighs and the activation in your glutes and quads.

Rise:

- Push through your heels to stand back up, straightening your legs. Squeeze your glutes at the top of the movement.
- Keep your chest up and core engaged throughout the entire movement.

Tips for Proper Form:

- **Avoid Leaning Forward**: Keep your chest up and back straight. Avoid leaning forward or rounding your back.
- **Control Your Movement**: Focus on a controlled descent and ascent. Avoid bouncing at the bottom of the squat.
- **Breathing**: Inhale as you lower your body, and exhale as you push back up to the starting position.

Modifications and Variations:

- **Dumbbell or Kettlebell**: For added resistance, hold a dumbbell or kettlebell with both hands in front of you (goblet style) during the squat.
- **Wide Stance**: Adjust the width of your stance to find the most comfortable and practical position for your body.
- **Depth Adjustment**: If you're new to sumo squats, start with a shallower squat and gradually increase your depth as you become more comfortable and flexible.

Advanced Variations on the Bicep Curl

Hammer Curl

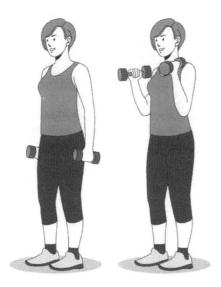

- **Setup:** Stand with your feet shoulder-width apart, holding a dumbbell in each hand with your palms facing your torso (neutral grip).

- **Performing the Curl:** Keep your upper arms at your sides and curl the weights while maintaining a neutral grip. Focus on engaging the brachialis muscle (located underneath the biceps).

- **Repetition:** Perform 8-12 reps for 2-3 sets.

Bicep 21 Curls

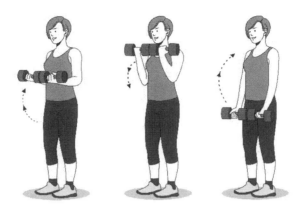

- **Setup:** Stand with your feet shoulder-width apart, holding a dumbbell in each hand with your palms facing forward.

- **Performing the Curl:**
    1. **For the first 7 reps,** Curl the weights from the starting position to halfway up (90-degree angle).
    2. **Next 7 reps:** Curl the weights from halfway up to the top position.
    3. **Last 7 reps:** Perform full-range curls from the starting position to the top.

Advanced Variation on the Row

Single-Arm Row

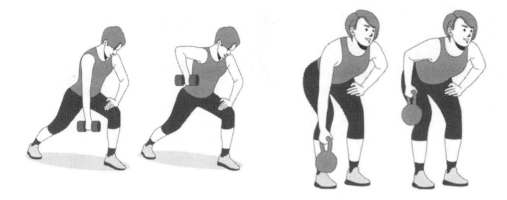

- **Setup:** Place your left knee and hand on a bench for support. Hold a weight in your right hand, letting it hang straight down.

- **Performing the Row:** Pull the weight toward your hip, keeping your elbow close to your body. Lower it back down with control.

- **Switch Sides:** Perform the same number of reps with the left arm.

- **Repetition:** Perform 8-12 reps for 2-3 sets on each arm.

Advanced Tips:

- **Focus on the Squeeze:** Hold the top position for a second or two to emphasize the contraction of your back muscles.
- **Increase the Challenge:** To make the exercise more difficult, use heavier weights, increase the number of repetitions, or add a pause at the top of the movement.
- **Engage Your Core:** Maintain a strong core throughout the exercise to protect your lower back and improve overall stability.

Following these instructions and tips, you can safely and effectively perform bent-over rows to strengthen your back and improve your upper body strength.

Advanced Variations on the Shoulder Press

Arnold Press

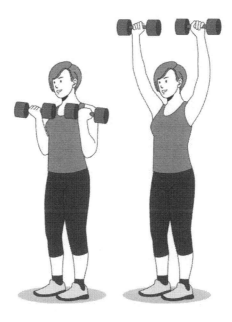

- **Setup:** Stand or sit with a dumbbell in each hand, starting with your palms facing your body and the dumbbells at shoulder height.

- **Performing the Press:** As you press the weights upward, rotate your palms to face forward. Reverse the motion as you lower the weights back down.

- **Repetition:** Perform 8-12 reps for 2-3 sets.

Single-Arm Dumbbell Shoulder Press

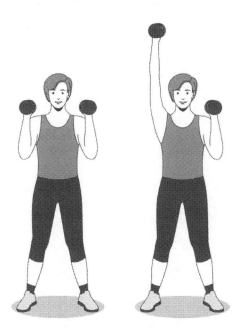

- **Setup:** Stand or sit with a dumbbell in one hand at shoulder height, using the other for balance if needed.

- **Performing the Press:** Press the dumbbell upward with one arm, then lower it back down. Switch arms after completing the desired reps.

- **Repetition:** Perform 8-12 reps for 2-3 sets on each arm.

Advanced Tips:

- **Increase the Challenge:** To increase the difficulty of the exercise, use heavier weights, increase the number of repetitions, or add a pause at the top of the movement.
- **Engage Your Core:** Maintain a strong core throughout the exercise to protect your lower back and improve overall stability.
- **Focus on Form:** Prioritize proper form over lifting heavier weights to reduce the risk of injury and maximize muscle engagement.

Following these instructions and tips, you can safely and effectively perform the dumbbell shoulder press to build strength and improve overall upper-body muscle definition.

Advanced Variations on the Glute Bridge

Single-leg Glute Bridge

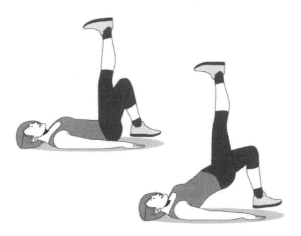

- **Setup:** Start in the standard glute bridge position.

- **Performing the Bridge:** Lift one leg off the ground, keeping it straight or bent, and perform the glute bridge with the other leg.

- **Switch Sides:** Complete the desired reps on one leg, then switch to the other leg.

- **Repetition:** Perform 8-12 reps per side for 2-3 sets.

Tips for Advanced Variations:

- **Start Slow:** Begin with lighter resistance or lower elevation if trying these variations for the first time.
- **Focus on Form:** Maintain proper form and core engagement, even with the added difficulty.
- **Gradual Progression:** Gradually increase the difficulty as your strength and stability improve.

By following these instructions and incorporating advanced variations, you can effectively perform the glute bridge exercise to strengthen your glutes, hamstrings, and lower back while improving overall hip mobility and core stability.

Advanced Variations on the Triceps Extension

Overhead Triceps Extension

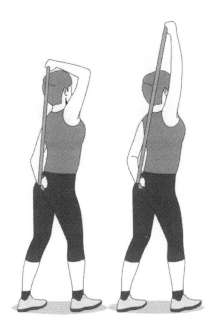

- **Setup:** Stand with your feet shoulder-width apart, holding a resistance band with both hands. Extend one arm straight above your head, keeping your elbows close to your ears.

- **Performing the Extension:** Inhale as you slowly release the tension on the band behind your head by bending your elbows. Exhale as you extend your arms back to the starting position, squeezing your triceps. This can also be done with a dumbbell.

- **Repetition:** Perform 10-15 reps for 2-3 sets.

Tips for Advanced Exercises:

- **Start with Lighter Weights:** If you're new to these advanced exercises, start with lighter weights to ensure proper form.
- **Focus on Form:** Maintain proper form throughout each exercise to avoid injury and maximize effectiveness.
- **Gradually Increase Weight:** As you become more comfortable with the exercises, gradually increase the weight to continue challenging your muscles.

Balance Enhancing Equipment:

Incorporating a Bosu ball into your workouts presents another excellent opportunity to challenge your balance further. With its unstable surface, the Bosu ball forces you to engage multiple muscle groups to maintain stability. Try performing squats or step-ups on the Bosu ball. When standing on the dome-shaped side, your body must adapt to the shifting balance, significantly improving your reflexes and core strength. These effective exercises inject a fun, playful element into your workout routine, keeping you engaged and eager to progress.

Using equipment like stability balls and balance boards can significantly enhance the effectiveness of your balance training. Stability balls, for example, can be used for various exercises that improve core strength and stability. Sitting on a stability ball and performing pelvic tilts or abdominal curls challenges your balance and deeply engages your core muscles. Balance boards, on the other hand, add an element of instability that makes even basic exercises like standing or squatting much more challenging. As you strive to maintain your balance on the board, you engage smaller, often underutilized muscles that play crucial roles in maintaining stability.

It is advisable to have something nearby that you can hold on to when gaining balance, whether using a Bosu balance board or stability ball. These are very advanced tools, and we want to build up to using them—but not at the risk of falling.

When integrated thoughtfully and progressively into your fitness routine, balance training can transform your daily move and feel. It's about more than just preventing falls; it's about empowering yourself to move confidently and live independently. Whether stepping onto a curb, reaching for an item on a high shelf, or playing with your grandchildren, enhanced balance and stability permeate every aspect of your life, allowing you to live fully and fearlessly.

6.3 Exploring High-intensity Low-impact Training (HILIT)

High-intensity Low-impact Training, or HILIT, is a delightful twist on traditional high-intensity workouts. It delivers all the robust benefits without the stress on your joints. Picture this: You're engaging in bursts of heart-pumping activity that boosts your cardiovascular health and accelerates calorie burning, but you're not subjecting your body to the pounding and jarring that come with high-impact exercises. This approach is perfect for those who want to protect their joints without compromising on the intensity needed to see significant health improvements.

Designing a HILIT session is both an art and a science. It involves structuring intervals of intense activity followed by periods of lower intensity or rest, allowing you to push your body to its aerobic limits without overburdening it. Typically, a session lasts 20 to 30 minutes and can be tailored to suit any fitness level. For instance, you might start with three minutes of fast walking or light jogging, followed by one minute of brisk walking. As you progress, you can introduce more varied exercises like cycling, swimming, or using an elliptical machine, adjusting the intensity and duration based on your comfort and improvement in fitness levels.

Let's dive into a sample HILIT routine that you can try, either at home or in a gym setting. Begin with a five-minute warm-up of gentle stretching and light cardio to increase your heart rate. Then, move into the core of the workout: alternate between one minute of intense activity, such as speed walking, stationary biking, or rowing and one minute of active recovery, which could involve slower-paced movements or complete rest. Repeat this cycle for 15-20 minutes, depending on your fitness level. To end, cool down with five minutes of slow walking and light stretching to help your muscles recover and prevent stiffness.

Monitoring the intensity of your workouts and ensuring adequate recovery can be done using a heart rate monitor or fitness tracker, which will help you know that you're working within your target heart rate zones, maximizing benefits while keeping an eye on your safety. These devices can help you see when you might be pushing too hard or not enough, allowing you to adjust your effort level in real-time.

Incorporating HILIT into your workout regimen opens up a new avenue to boost your fitness without compromising joint health. Its adaptability makes it a suitable and effective workout choice, whether just starting your fitness journey or looking to shake up an established routine. As you explore HILIT, remember to listen to your body, adjust the intensity as needed, and enjoy getting fit in a way that respects and protects your body's needs.

6.4 Progressive Overload: What It Is and How to Use It

Progressive overload is not just a fancy term tossed around in fitness circles; it's the cornerstone of effective strength training, especially as we age. The concept is straightforward: continuously challenge your muscles by increasing their demands over time. This method ensures your muscles don't become complacent; they must adapt, grow, and strengthen in response to these increased demands. Think of it as a gentle but firm nudge to encourage your body to enhance its capacity. This approach is crucial because you might hit a plateau without it, seeing no meaningful improvement despite regular workouts.

There are various ways to implement progressive overload in your routine, and the key is to find methods that suit your current fitness level and overall health. One straightforward method is to increase the weight you lift. Adding even a small amount of weight to your exercises forces your muscles to work harder than they're accustomed to. Another technique is altering your repetition counts. If you're used to performing ten reps of a particular exercise, pushing yourself for one or two additional reps can significantly enhance the training stimulus, promoting muscle growth and endurance.

Weightlifting with increasing weight and decreasing reps, known as progressive overload, aims to build strength and muscle. Here's how it works:

- Choose a weight you can lift for 8-12 reps.
- Gradually increase the weight in subsequent sets or sessions.
- As the weight increases, decrease the number of reps (e.g., from 8-12 to 4-6 reps).
- Maintain proper form to prevent injury.
- Allow adequate rest (1-2 minutes) between sets for recovery.

Changing the tempo of your exercises can also create a new challenge for your muscles. For instance, slowing down the pace at which you perform an exercise can increase the time your muscles are under tension. This change forces them to adapt and grow stronger. For example, when performing a squat, try lowering yourself slowly to a count of three, hold at the bottom for two seconds, and then push back up to a count of three. This method increases muscle strength and enhances your control and stability during the exercise.

Adjusting the principles of progressive overload to suit age and individual fitness levels is particularly important. Our bodies require more recovery time as we age, and our joints might be more susceptible to strain. Therefore, it's important to challenge our muscles and acknowledge and respect our body's signals. Start with lighter weights and fewer repetitions, focusing on maintaining perfect form to prevent injuries. Gradually increase the intensity of your workouts, and always prioritize quality over quantity. If you experience pain or discomfort beyond normal muscle fatigue, take it as a sign to scale back and reassess your approach.

So, as you plan your next workout, consider how you can gently increase the demands on your body to keep your muscles guessing and growing. Remember, the goal is gradual improvement, ensuring that each step you take is toward greater strength and vitality.

6.5 Leveraging Technology for Enhanced Training

In today's digital age, technology has seamlessly integrated into almost every aspect of our lives, and fitness is no exception. Embracing technology in your fitness regime can significantly enhance the quality and effectiveness of your workouts, providing you with tools that were once accessible only in professional settings. From fitness apps that help design workouts to wearable technology that monitors your physical activity, the options are vast and can be tailored to your personal fitness goals and preferences.

Fitness apps are particularly beneficial, as they make it seem like a personal trainer is in your pocket. These apps can guide you through various workouts, whether at home or in the gym, with detailed instructions and videos to ensure you perform each exercise correctly. Many apps also offer workout customization based on your fitness level and the equipment you have available, making them a versatile tool for anyone looking to enhance their strength training routine. For instance, apps like MyFitnessPal track your workouts and help you monitor your diet, which is crucial for overall health and fitness. Others, like Nike Training Club, provide various workout plans that can adapt to your evolving fitness levels and goals. Using these apps, you can maintain a well-rounded fitness routine that supports your strength training endeavors and helps you stay on track with your health objectives.

Wearable technology, such as activity trackers and heart rate monitors, takes your training to the next level by providing real-time feedback on your physical activities. These devices can monitor your heart rate, count steps, track sleep patterns, and even analyze your body's response to different exercises. By wearing a Fitbit, Oura Ring, or an Apple Watch, you can get instant feedback on how hard you work during each session and ensure you stay within safe heart rate zones. Additionally, seeing the data can be incredibly motivating; it's rewarding to see the tangible results of your efforts, such as calories burned or improvements in heart health over time.

Online training programs offer another fantastic way to diversify your workout routine. These programs, often led by certified trainers, provide structured workouts that can be accessed from anywhere with an internet connection and help keep your fitness front of mind, even when traveling. Platforms like Peloton or Daily Burn deliver various workout styles, from high-intensity interval training to yoga and Pilates, catering to different fitness levels and interests. These programs often include community features, allowing you to connect with other users for support. By participating in these online programs, you can experience the guidance of a personal trainer and the dynamic atmosphere of a class, all from the comfort of your home.

As we conclude this chapter on leveraging technology for enhanced training, we've explored how modern tools can significantly enrich your fitness routine. From the convenience and customization offered by fitness apps to the motivating real-time data from wearable technology and the engaging experiences provided by online programs and virtual classes, technology has opened up new and exciting avenues for maintaining and enhancing our fitness. These tools support our physical health and encourage us to stay connected and motivated as we pursue our fitness journeys.

The next chapter will examine the health and wellness practices that support your strength training journey, ensuring you have a holistic approach to fitness that encompasses not just physical strength but also overall wellbeing.

7

Connecting the Mind and Body

Imagine your body as a symphony orchestra. Each section, from strings to percussion, plays a role, but without a conductor to guide them, the music might lack harmony and direction. Similarly, in strength training, your body performs the physical work, but your mind acts as the conductor, ensuring every move is purposeful and harmonized. This chapter explores the profound relationship between mind and body, mainly through practices like mindfulness and meditation that can enhance your strength training, enrich your mental focus, and deepen the connection to your body's movements.

7.1 Mindfulness and Meditation for Strength Trainers

Integrating mindfulness into your strength training routine is akin to tuning an instrument before a performance—it ensures you are fully present and can deliver your best. The essence of mindfulness in fitness involves focusing intently on your body's movements, the rhythm of your breath, and the sensations you experience during each exercise. This attentive state can transform routine workouts into a rich, engaging process, enhancing both the efficiency and enjoyment of your training.

Begin by incorporating breath control into your exercises. For example, when performing a bicep curl, inhale as you lower the weights, feel the air fill your lungs, and exhale as you lift, tuning into the muscle tension. This helps maintain a rhythmic pace and increases awareness of your body's mechanics and responses. Similarly, during a squat, focus on the alignment of your knees, the distribution of weight on your feet, and the strength in your core. Such mindfulness can prevent injuries and promote more effective muscle engagement.

Post-workout meditation can be a powerful tool for enhancing recovery and decreasing stress levels. After your muscles have been activated and challenged, sitting quietly and meditating can help shift your body into rest and recovery. Simple techniques like guided imagery, where you visualize a peaceful scene, or progressive muscle relaxation, where you tense and relax different muscle groups, can significantly reduce physical tension and mental stress. This deliberate slowing down allows your body to initiate repair processes more efficiently and deepens your well-being.

The concept of mindful repetitions is another transformative practice. Instead of counting repetitions merely as numbers, focus on the quality and feeling of each movement. For instance, imagine drawing energy up from the ground through your feet and legs with each lift, channeling it through your core. This visualization enhances your mental engagement and connects you more deeply with the exercise, potentially increasing its effectiveness.

Setting intentions before your workout can also profoundly impact your physical performance and mental clarity. Before you start, take a moment to articulate a clear, positive intention for your session. It could be as straightforward as, "Today, I will focus on maintaining form," or more reflective, such as, "I will honor my body's strengths and limits." This practice prepares you mentally and emotionally and aligns your physical energy with your mental focus, creating a more holistic workout experience.

Mindful Breathing Exercise
Try this simple breathing technique to cultivate mindfulness during your next workout:

1. Find a comfortable, seated position with your legs crossed. You can sit on a folded blanket or yoga bolster if that is more comfortable. It is also not necessary to fold your feet over your thighs.
2. Close your eyes and take a deep breath through your nose, counting to four.
3. Hold your breath for a count of seven.
4. Exhale slowly through your mouth for a count of eight.
5. Repeat this cycle four times.

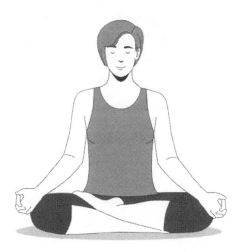

This exercise helps regulate your breathing and centers your mind, making it easier to maintain focus during strength training. It's a valuable tool that enhances your workouts and improves overall well-being by reducing stress and increasing mental clarity.

By weaving mindfulness and meditation into your strength training, you enhance your physical endurance and muscle strength, cultivating a deeper, more rewarding connection with your body. This holistic approach transforms your workouts into more meaningful sessions and contributes significantly to your overall health and mental well-being. As you continue to practice these techniques, your training sessions will become about physical fitness, personal growth, and inner balance.

7.2 The Psychological Benefits of Regular Exercise

When we consider the impact of regular exercise, we often think of visible changes in our physical appearance or capabilities. However, strength training, particularly as you navigate the later chapters of your life, holds profound psychological benefits that can be just as transformative as the physical ones. Understanding how regular physical activity influences mental health can provide additional motivation and appreciation for your workout routine.

One of exercise's most immediate mental benefits is the release of endorphins, often known as the body's natural "feel-good" chemicals. Strength training triggers these biochemicals in your brain, which act as natural painkillers and mood elevators. This endorphin boost, or the "runner's high," is not exclusive to running; lifting weights or performing resistance exercises can elicit the same euphoric reaction. The lift in mood following a workout session is more than merely anecdotal. Scientific studies support that even moderate physical activity can stimulate endorphin release, helping to elevate your mood immediately. For you, this might mean feeling a noticeable decrease in stress levels and noticing a buoyant sense of well-being after your training sessions, making the exercises not just a physical challenge but a delightful mood enhancer.

Beyond the biochemical effects, regular engagement in strength training can significantly enhance your self-esteem and body image. Achieving your fitness goals, whether lifting heavier weights, mastering a new exercise, or simply being consistent in your routine, translates into a profound sense of accomplishment. This success breeds confidence, not just in your physical abilities but in your overall self-worth. Your body image tends to improve as you grow stronger and see tangible results from your efforts. You start to see yourself as capable and strong, which can be incredibly empowering, especially in a society that often undervalues older adults.

The role of regular exercise in managing and reducing symptoms of anxiety and depression has also been well-documented. Engaging in strength training can act as a powerful counterbalance to these conditions. Physical activity helps to regulate the neurotransmitters serotonin and dopamine in your brain, similar to the effects of some antidepressant medications. Furthermore, the structured nature of a workout regimen can provide a comforting routine, often serving as a therapeutic break from the stressors of daily life. For many, the gym or home workout space becomes a sanctuary where you can shed your anxieties and focus solely on your physical movements and the strength of your body.

Lastly, the cognitive benefits of regular physical activity are profound and particularly relevant as you age. Studies have shown that exercise can enhance cognitive function and improve memory, attention, and problem-solving skills. This mental boost is believed to result from increased blood flow to the brain during physical activity, which nourishes your brain cells with oxygen and nutrients and may help form new neuronal connections. The focus and concentration required to perform and maintain various strength training exercises also promote mental clarity, making each session a brain workout.

The psychological benefits of strength training create a compelling case for making exercise a regular part of your life. Not only are you sculpting a more muscular body, but you are also fostering a resilient and vibrant mind. Each workout session is an opportunity to enhance your physical health and elevate your mental state, proving that strength training is a holistic approach to wellness. As you continue to engage in your fitness routine, remember that every rep strengthens your muscles and fortifies your mental health, solidifying the profound connection between your mind and body.

7.3 Stress Reduction through Physical Activity

Engaging in physical activity is more than a method for improving physical fitness; it's a potent tool for stress management. When you exercise, your body undergoes a series of physiological changes that collectively help decrease stress levels. One of the primary mechanisms at work is the reduction of stress hormones, such as cortisol and adrenaline. These hormones, which are crucial in the 'fight or flight' response, can be overstimulated during prolonged periods of stress, leading to feelings of anxiety and restlessness. Regular physical activity prompts your body to moderate the release of these hormones, helping to maintain a calmer, more balanced state.

Moreover, exercise stimulates the production of endorphins—chemicals in the brain that act as natural painkillers and mood elevators. This biochemical process is crucial not only immediately following exercise but also in building long-term resilience against stress. Activities particularly effective in this regard include rhythmic, repetitive exercises such as walking, cycling, or swimming. These activities help establish a meditative-like state that fosters calmness and helps dissipate stress, providing a double benefit and enhancing physical health.

Creating a relaxing workout environment can further enhance the stress-reducing effects of exercise. Consider the atmosphere in which you engage in physical activity; it can significantly affect how you perceive and benefit from your workout. Simple adjustments like playing soothing music can profoundly affect your mood and stress levels. Music has been shown to lower cortisol levels and enhance feelings of relaxation. Similarly, incorporating elements of aromatherapy, such as diffusing calming essential oils like lavender or chamomile in your workout space, can create a serene atmosphere that not only makes the environment more pleasant but also physically helps to reduce stress through the olfactory impact on the brain.

Another powerful aspect of using exercise as a stress management tool is the routine it establishes in your daily life. Regular exercise schedules provide a sense of predictability and control that is often lacking in a chaotic life. This routine creates a structure that can be incredibly reassuring, offering a consistent time and space dedicated to caring for your body and mind. It becomes a ritual, a respite from the day's stresses, and a committed time when you can disconnect from external pressures. The predictability of a routine can significantly ease anxiety, as familiarity and repetition provide a comforting and dependable break from unpredictability and stress.

By embracing these strategies, you actively enhance your body's ability to manage stress, not just temporarily but as a part of a sustained lifestyle change. Regular physical activity becomes a powerful ally in maintaining mental health, and by creating a supportive, pleasant exercise environment and sticking to a routine, you harness even greater benefits from your fitness endeavors. This holistic approach does not merely seek to improve physical fitness but aims to enrich your quality of life by fostering a resilient, stress-resistant mindset. Through these practices, you can transform your exercise routine into a powerful tool for managing stress and enhancing your physical and mental health in profound and lasting ways.

7.4 Yoga and Pilates: Complementary Practices for Strength Training

In fitness, diversity in your exercise regimen isn't just beneficial; it's essential for fostering a well-rounded approach to health. Yoga and Pilates, often revered for their calming and restorative properties, are not merely about stretching or achieving a peaceful state of mind. These practices are powerhouse activities that can significantly enhance your strength training efforts by improving flexibility, balance, and core stability. Let's delve into how these gentle yet formidable practices can complement your strength training and contribute to a holistic approach to your physical health.

Yoga, with its diverse range of postures and sequences, provides an excellent complement to strength training. Each pose in yoga increases flexibility and balance. For instance, poses like the Warrior series improve leg strength, enhance stability, and increase hip flexibility, which is beneficial for compound exercises like squats and lunges in your regular workouts. Moreover, yoga's emphasis on flexibility can help alleviate the muscle stiffness and tightness often associated with weightlifting, enhancing your range of motion and reducing the risk of injuries. The balance poses in yoga, such as Tree Pose, require a deep focus and physical steadiness that aid in developing the small stabilizing muscles. These muscles help maintain proper posture and alignment during your lifts, ensuring you perform each exercise effectively and safely.

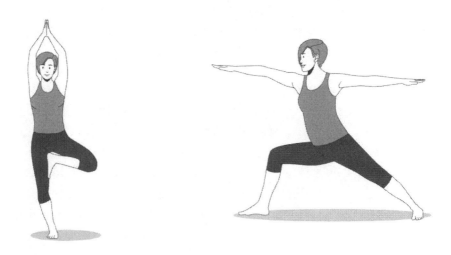

Tree Pose   **Warrior Pose**

Pilates also emphasizes proper alignment and core engagement with every movement. An engaged core translates directly into better core performance during your strength training routines. For example, an essential Pilates exercise like the 'Hundred' fires up your core muscles and teaches you to coordinate your breath with muscle contractions—skills invaluable when performing core-intensive strength exercises such as deadlifts or overhead presses. By enhancing your core strength and stability, Pilates ensures you can handle heavier weights and more complex movements in your strength training, leading to better overall muscle growth and toning.

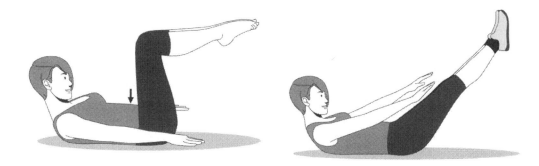

The Hundred can be done with the legs bent or straight and even with the feet on the floor if you are starting. The movement is:

Lift:
- Raise your head, neck, and shoulders off the mat. Your gaze should be toward your navel.
- Extend your legs to a 45-degree angle from the floor. You can keep your knees bent at a 90-degree angle if this is too challenging.

Arm Movement:
- Lift your arms off the floor to about shoulder height.
- Pump your arms up and down with small, controlled movements, keeping them straight and parallel to the floor.

Breathing:
- Inhale for five counts, then exhale for five counts.
- Repeat this cycle for ten sets, totaling 100 arm pumps.

Modifications:
- **Neck Support**: If you feel strain in your neck, you can keep your head on the floor or use a small cushion for support.
- **Leg Position**: For beginners, you can keep your knees bent at a 90-degree angle or place your feet on the floor.

Finishing:
- **Lower Down**: After completing the Hundred, gently lower your head, shoulders, and legs back to the starting position.

Integrating yoga and Pilates into your weekly training schedule can be refreshing and strategically beneficial. Consider dedicating at least two weekly sessions to these practices, ideally when not engaging in strength training. This scheduling allows your body to recover from the strenuous demands of lifting while still staying active and working on essential fitness components like flexibility, balance, and core strength.

7.5 The Power of Positive Thinking in Fitness

In fitness, cultivating a positive mindset can transform your workout routine from a chore into a delightful part of your day, making each session more successful and enjoyable.

One effective strategy to foster a positive mindset is to focus on the reasons behind your fitness efforts. Remind yourself regularly why you are committed to staying active. It could be the desire to play with your grandchildren without feeling winded or about managing a health condition more effectively. Keeping these motivating factors at the forefront of your mind can transform your attitude toward working out from seeing it as a burden to viewing it as a valuable tool for a happier, healthier life. Additionally, celebrate every small victory along the way. Did you lift heavier weights this week than last week?

Did you complete your workout despite not feeling up to it? Recognizing these significant accomplishments can boost your morale and reinforce a positive mindset. Every time you show up for a workout, you are succeeding in prioritizing your health.

Affirmations and positive self-talk reinforce your visualization practices and help combat negative thoughts. Challenge demoralizing thoughts by transforming them into affirmations like, "Every workout makes me stronger and more capable." Repeat these affirmations daily, ideally in the morning or before your workouts. Moreover, affirmations can reshape your self-perception, making you more resilient against setbacks and more persistent in pursuing your fitness goals.

Here are some additional affirmations you might try:

"I am strong, capable, and becoming healthier with every workout."

- Remind yourself that each session strengthens you and contributes to your goals.

"My body deserves this care and attention; I honor it with every exercise."

- Recognize that strength training is a form of self-care, showing respect and love for your body.

"Age is just a number; I can build strength and confidence at any stage of life."

- Embrace the idea that it's never too late to start or continue improving your physical fitness.

"I am proud of my progress and excited for the journey ahead."

- Celebrate the achievements you've made, no matter how small, and look forward to future improvements.

"I am investing in my future health and independence by staying active and strong."

- Focus on the long-term benefits of strength training, such as maintaining independence and enjoying a high quality of life.

By adopting these approaches—celebrating small victories, challenging negative thoughts, using visualization, and practicing positive affirmations—you nurture a mindset that makes your workouts more enjoyable and enhances your overall perseverance and success in fitness.

7.6 Building Mental Resilience through Routine Exercise

Routine strength training does more than sculpt your body; it builds a fortress of mental resilience that can shield you through life's ups and downs. When you engage regularly in this physical discipline, you're not just lifting weights but also lifting your spirits and enhancing your ability to handle whatever life throws your way. Pushing through a challenging set or adding just one more rep can instill a profound sense of personal mastery and control. This isn't just about power over the weight; it's about claiming power over your life's circumstances.

Each time you complete a workout, you reinforce a message to yourself: You are capable, can handle challenges, and can exert control over your health and well-being. This sense of mastery is a critical component of psychological resilience, serving as a mental muscle that strengthens with each workout. Just as your physical muscles recover and grow stronger after being stressed, your mental resilience builds when you push through the challenges of a strenuous workout. This resilience spills over into other areas of your life, equipping you with the mental fortitude to tackle problems, handle stress more effectively, and recover from setbacks more quickly.

Building a supportive community within your fitness endeavors can significantly amplify your resilience. Joining a fitness class, participating in a lifting group, or even engaging with online communities of like-minded individuals can provide guidance, motivation, and emotional support. Communities can boost your commitment to your fitness goals and provide a safety net when you face setbacks, ensuring minor hiccups don't derail your long-term objectives. The long-term mental health benefits of sustained physical activity are profound.

As this chapter closes, remember that each time you lift a weight, you're not just training your muscles; you're training your mind to be stronger, more resilient, and more equipped to handle the complexities of life.

8

Long-term Health and Wellness

In this chapter, we'll explore how regular exercise can be a dynamic tool for managing chronic conditions such as diabetes, heart disease, and arthritis and how you can tailor your exercise program to work harmoniously with your medical treatments and lifestyle.

8.1 Managing Chronic Conditions with Regular Exercise

Exercise as Medicine

It's proven that regular physical activity can significantly prevent and manage various chronic conditions. Strength training, in particular, can be a potent medicine. For instance, it improves insulin sensitivity and enhances glucose metabolism—crucial for managing diabetes. For those dealing with heart disease, strength training helps maintain a healthy weight, lower blood pressure, and improve lipid profiles. For people living with arthritis, it strengthens the muscles around the joints, which reduces joint stress and alleviates pain.

But how exactly does this work? When you engage in strength training, your muscles get stronger and release a cascade of health-promoting hormones and chemicals that can help reduce inflammation, improve your body's use of insulin, and enhance your overall metabolism. These biological changes are powerful, particularly for those managing chronic diseases where inflammation and metabolic health are often significant issues.

Tailored Exercise Programs

Creating an exercise program that caters to your chronic condition involves careful planning and consideration. Let's take arthritis as an example. Low-impact exercises that improve the range of motion and strengthen muscles without putting undue stress on the joints can be particularly beneficial. Water aerobics, for example, can be a great choice, as the buoyancy of water reduces stress on joint surfaces while providing resistance that helps build muscle strength.

A combination of moderate-intensity aerobic exercises, like brisk walking or cycling, supplemented with two to three strength training sessions per week can be effective for combatting heart disease. The key is to start slowly and gradually increase the intensity of workouts as your body adapts and your fitness improves.

For those managing diabetes, consistency in exercise timing can also help regulate blood glucose levels more effectively. Incorporating activities you enjoy ensures that the routine is sustainable and adaptable to your daily life, which is crucial for long-term management.

For instance, if you're taking medications that affect your heart rate, your doctor may advise you to monitor your heart rate closely during exercise or may recommend safer specific exercise types. Similarly, if you have diabetes and use insulin, you'll need to understand how to adjust your insulin dosage on days you exercise to prevent hypoglycemia.

8.2 The Lifelong Benefits of Maintaining Muscle Mass

When we talk about aging gracefully, maintaining muscle mass plays a crucial role, much like the foundations of a house supporting its structure over the years. Sarcopenia, the age-related loss of muscle mass and strength, affects many of us as we age. However, engaging in regular strength training can effectively counteract this decline. Think of your muscles as allies that keep you moving and capable, supporting everything from lifting groceries to playing with grandchildren. By strengthening these allies, you combat the natural erosion of muscle mass and boost your body's overall functionality and resilience.

Muscle-building, or hypertrophy, involves creating small tears in muscle fibers through exercise. Your body repairs these tears and, in doing so, makes the fibers thicker and stronger. This natural response increases muscle mass and enhances your metabolic rate—the rate at which your body burns calories. Enhanced muscle mass means your body burns more calories, even at rest, helping you manage your weight and energy levels better. This metabolic boost is a critical factor in maintaining a healthy body weight and preventing obesity-related diseases such as type 2 diabetes and heart disease, which tend to become more prevalent as we age.

Moreover, the independence gained from a more muscular physique is significant. With increased muscle strength, daily activities like climbing stairs, carrying pets, or even simple tasks like opening jars become easier. This enhanced ability to perform everyday activities without assistance is what we refer to as functional independence. Maintaining this level of autonomy is not only crucial for physical health but also for mental wellbeing. It fosters a sense of self-efficacy and confidence, which can tremendously empower women, who often fear losing independence as they age.

Numerous studies support the correlation between muscular strength and longevity. A robust musculature is linked with reduced mortality rates, primarily because strong muscles improve mobility, balance, and recovery from illnesses or injuries. Moreover, the psychological benefits of maintaining an active lifestyle, characterized by regular strength training, contribute to improved quality of life. Individuals who engage in such activities report lower levels of anxiety and depression, better sleep patterns, and a more vibrant social life due to increased physical capabilities.

Building and maintaining muscle mass through strength training offers a cascade of benefits that enhance your metabolic health, functional independence, and overall quality of life. It allows you to lead a more active, autonomous, and enjoyable life, proving that age, while a number, does not define your capacity for vitality and vigor. As we continue to explore the multifaceted benefits of strength training, remember that each session is an investment not just in your physical health but also in a richer, more engaging life experience.

8.3 Preventing Falls and Injuries through Targeted Exercises

Falls and injuries, particularly among seniors, are not just minor setbacks but can significantly impact quality of life and independence. Imagine how a simple routine to strengthen your balance and coordination could transform your confidence, keeping you active and safe in your daily activities. By incorporating specific exercises into your regimen, you can significantly reduce the risk of falls, ensuring you continue to enjoy a vibrant, active lifestyle without fear.

Balance and Coordination Training

Integrating these exercises into your daily routine can be a manageable time commitment. Spending just a few minutes each day on these activities can lead to noticeable improvements in your stability. As your confidence grows, so does your ability to easily perform various daily tasks, from navigating stairs to walking on uneven surfaces. The key is consistency; similar to tuning an instrument regularly to keep it playing beautifully, regular practice of balance exercises keeps your body's reflexes sharp and responsive.

Strength Exercises for Injury Prevention

Now, let's focus on strengthening exercises targeting the muscles and joints most vulnerable to injuries—hips, knees, and ankles. By fortifying these areas, you can create a robust defense against the strains or sprains that often accompany falls. Exercises like squats and lunges are fantastic for building strength in your legs and hips. They enhance muscle mass and improve flexibility, making you less susceptible to injuries from sudden movements or falls. For added safety, consider performing these exercises using a chair for support, ensuring you can maintain proper form without risking a fall.

Resistance training can also be highly effective. Light weights or resistance bands can help strengthen smaller muscle groups that play crucial roles in joint stability. Calf raises, for instance, strengthen the lower leg muscles, which support ankle stability, while hip abductor exercises help protect your hips. When performed regularly, these exercises ensure that your joints are supported by strong muscles, significantly reducing the risk of injury.

Listening to your body is the most important strategy for adjusting your exercise routine to avoid injury. Pay attention to how your body feels during and after workouts. If you notice persistent pain or fatigue, it might be a sign that you're pushing too hard or that an aspect of your routine isn't working for your body anymore. On the other hand, feeling energized and strong after a workout indicates that your balance of activity, rest, and recovery is on point.

Heightened awareness and responsiveness to your body's signals are key in adapting your workouts effectively. They help prevent overtraining, reduce the risk of injury, and ensure that your exercise regimen genuinely contributes to your overall wellbeing and quality of life. Remember, each person's body is unique, and what works for one might not work for another. Therefore, stay attuned to your physical cues and be willing to adjust your activities accordingly.

This approach keeps you safe and makes your fitness routine a more enjoyable and rewarding part of your life as you age.

8.4 Planning for a Healthy Future: Beyond Strength Training

Integrating a variety of physical activities into your lifestyle ensures that your fitness routine remains engaging and contributes to a well-rounded health profile. Imagine weaving in activities such as swimming, cycling, or even dance classes alongside your strength training sessions. Each activity brings unique benefits, working different muscle groups, improving cardiovascular health, and boosting mental health through varied social interactions and environments.

The realm of health and fitness is ever-evolving, with new research and trends continuously emerging. Embracing the concept of lifelong learning within this field can significantly enhance your wellbeing. Staying informed about the latest research fuels your intellectual curiosity and empowers you to make educated decisions about your health. This might involve subscribing to health newsletters, attending workshops, or participating in community health talks. This ongoing education helps you adapt your fitness strategy based on the latest findings, ensuring your approach remains effective and aligned with current health standards.

Regular health screenings and check-ups are vital in monitoring your health status, especially as you age. These check-ups provide a snapshot of your health, offering insights to help you tailor your fitness routines. For instance, bone density scans, blood pressure checks, and cholesterol levels can influence the exercise you focus on. Regular screenings can catch potential health issues early, allowing for prompt and effective management. Discussing these results with your healthcare provider during routine visits ensures that your exercise regimen complements any medical treatments or dietary requirements, maintaining a holistic approach to your health.

Maintaining an active lifestyle does more than keep you fit; it sets a powerful example for your family and friends, inspiring them to prioritize their health. This legacy of health is one of the most valuable inheritances you can pass on to future generations. It teaches resilience, the importance of self-care, and the joy of active living. When family members see the tangible benefits of your fitness routine—your increased energy, enhanced mobility, and positive outlook—they are encouraged to embrace a more active lifestyle. This ripple effect can foster a culture of health and wellness within your community, contributing to a healthier, happier society.

These strategies—embracing various physical activities, committing to lifelong learning, staying on top of health screenings, and inspiring others through your fitness journey—ensure that your approach to health and wellness is balanced, informed, and influential. By incorporating these elements into your life, you enhance your health and inspire those around you, creating a lasting impact that transcends the immediate benefits of fitness.

Encourage and Support Other Women

Now you have everything you need to start and achieve your strength training goals, it's time to pass on your newfound knowledge and show other readers where they can find the same help.

By leaving your honest opinion of this book on Amazon, you'll show other midlife women looking to discover the true benefits of strength training where they can find the information they're looking for and develop their passion for strength training.

I appreciate your help. Information is kept alive when we pass on our knowledge – and you're helping us to do just that.

Scan the QR code below to leave your review on Amazon:

Conclusion

Let's take a moment to reflect on the transformative path we've embarked upon together. Starting or continuing strength training can significantly alter your life physically and in every facet. It's about building and preserving muscle mass, enhancing bone density, and boosting vitality. More than that, it fosters a sense of independence that can redefine this beautiful chapter of your life.

Strength training transcends the physical; it's a holistic practice that nurtures your mental and emotional well-being. It reduces stress, improves mental health, and forges a strong sense of belonging through community. Remember, this is not just about lifting weights; it's about lifting each other and sharing experiences and strength in more ways than one.

I want to remind you that strength training is incredibly adaptable. No matter your starting point or the unique challenges, there's always a way to tailor exercises and routines to meet your needs. This adaptability ensures you can enjoy the benefits of strength training, making it a perfect fit for your lifestyle and capabilities.

The importance of a supportive community cannot be overstated. Whether through local classes, vibrant online communities, or simply involving your family in your fitness journey, the encouragement and motivation from others are invaluable. These connections help you stick with your regimen and make the activities enjoyable and deeply rewarding.

As you age gracefully, it is crucial to embrace lifelong learning and adaptability in your approach to fitness. Stay curious and informed about new research and trends in health and wellness that can enhance your routines and overall well-being. Don't shy away from adjusting your exercises as your body needs to evolve.

Let me urge you to take that first step today if you haven't already. It's never too late to start reaping the myriad benefits of strength training. Imagine the profound impact it can have on your health, your confidence, and your quality of life. Start small, celebrate every progress, and set new, achievable goals. Keep pushing forward, always striving for a healthier, more vibrant future.

Share your journey—inspire others! Whether through social media, blogging, or chatting with friends and family, your story can motivate someone to start their journey toward better health.

As we conclude, remember that strength training is a path of self-discovery and empowerment. It promises lasting health benefits and a journey filled with achievements. Take this book as your guide and companion along the way. Revisit it whenever you need a reminder of how far you've come and how much further you can go.

Thank you for allowing me to be a part of your fitness journey. Let's continue striving for strength, health, and a joyful heart together. Here's to lifting more than weights—here's to lifting spirits and building a thriving, supportive community of strong women not held back by the natural process of aging.

References

1. Alloy. (n.d.). Why strength training for women is crucial as you age. Alloy Franchise. https://alloyfranchise.com/blog/strength-training-for-women-as-age/

2. Art of Manliness. (n.d.). How to build a home gym on the cheap. Art of Manliness. https://www.artofmanliness.com/health-fitness/fitness/how-to-build-a-home-gym-on-the-cheap/

3. KS Body Shop. (n.d.). Meet 2 older superwomen who prove the power of fitness. KS Body Shop. https://ksbodyshop.com/success-story-older-superwomen-who-prove-power-of-fitness/

4. Mayo Clinic. (n.d.). How fit are you? See how you measure up. Mayo Clinic. https://www.mayoclinic.org/healthy-lifestyle/fitness/in-depth/fitness/art-20046433

5. WebMD. (n.d.). Strength training for your rheumatoid arthritis. WebMD. https://www.webmd.com/rheumatoid-arthritis/features/strength-exercises-for-ra

6. National Center for Biotechnology Information. (n.d.). The role of high-intensity and high-impact exercises in... https://www.ncbi.nlm.nih.gov/pmc/articles/PMC9990535/

7. National Center for Biotechnology Information. (n.d.). Effects of resistance exercise on bone health. https://www.ncbi.nlm.nih.gov/pmc/articles/PMC6279907/

8. Harvard Health. (n.d.). The best core exercises for older adults. Harvard Health. https://www.health.harvard.edu/staying-healthy/the-best-core-exercises-for-older-adults

9. Stanford Center on Longevity. (2024, January 23). Protein needs for adults 50+. Healthful Nutrition. https://longevity.stanford.edu/lifestyle/2024/01/23/protein-needs-for-adults-50/

10. Precision Hydration. (n.d.). Should your hydration strategy change as you get older? Precision Hydration. https://www.precisionhydration.com/performance-advice/hydration/should-your-hydration-strategy-change-as-you-get-older/

11. Abbott Nutrition News. (n.d.). Muscle recovery: A key component to healthy aging. Abbott Nutrition News. https://www.nutritionnews.abbott/healthy-living/aging-well/Muscle-Recovery-A-Key-Component-to-Healthy-Aging/

12. Ageist. (n.d.). Doctor-recommended over-50 exercise and recovery program. Ageist. https://www.ageist.com/wellness/health/doctor-recommended-over-50-exercise-and-recovery-program/

13. Verywell Fit. (n.d.). Strength training for seniors: A 20-minute workout. Verywell Fit. https://www.verywellfit.com/20-minute-senior-weight-training-workout-3498676

14. Cleveland Clinic. (n.d.). How SMART fitness goals can help you get healthier. Cleveland Clinic. https://health.clevelandclinic.org/smart-fitness-goals

15. Health.com. (n.d.). Combining strength training and cardio may help longevity. Health.com. https://www.health.com/combining-strength-training-cardio-longevity-6748178

16. LIT Method. (n.d.). 10 resistance band workouts for seniors. LIT Method. https://www.lit-method.com/blogs/boltcut-blog/resistance-band-exercises-for-seniors

17. Tonal. (n.d.). How to do high-intensity, low-impact exercise. Tonal. https://www.to-nal.com/blog/high-intensity-low-impact-exercise/

18. National Center for Biotechnology Information. (n.d.). Initiating and maintaining resistance training in older adults. https://www.ncbi.nlm.nih.gov/pmc/articles/PMC2709760/

19. SilverSneakers. (n.d.). 8 best fitness apps for older adults. SilverSneakers. https://www.silversneakers.com/blog/8-best-fitness-apps-for-older-adults/

20. National Center for Biotechnology Information. (n.d.). Mindfulness-based interventions for older adults. https://www.ncbi.nlm.nih.gov/pmc/articles/PMC4868399/

21. National Center for Biotechnology Information. (n.d.). The effect of resistance training on health-related quality. https://www.ncbi.nlm.nih.gov/pmc/articles/PMC6377696/

22. Man Flow Yoga. (n.d.). Creating a combined yoga and strength training routine. Man Flow Yoga. https://manflowyoga.com/blog/creating-a-combined-yoga-and-strength-training-routine/

23. Human Kinetics. (n.d.). Confidence and positive attitude help older adults stick with exercise. Human Kinetics. https://us.humankinetics.com/blogs/excerpt/confidence-and-positive-attitude-help-older-adults-stick-with-exercise

24. BMC Geriatrics. (n.d.). Regular group exercise contributes to balanced health in... https://bmcgeriatr.biomedcentral.com/articles/10.1186/s12877-017-0584-3

25. Senior Planet. (n.d.). Virtual fitness and wellness classes. Senior Planet. https://senior-planet.org/virtual-fitness-wellness-events/

26. Next Avenue. (n.d.). 9 volunteer jobs that could boost your health. Next Avenue. https://www.nextavenue.org/volunteer-jobs-boost-health/

27. National Institute on Aging. (n.d.). How can strength training build healthier bodies as we age? National Institute on Aging. https://www.nia.nih.gov/news/how-can-strength-training-build-healthier-bodies-we-age

28. Centers for Disease Control and Prevention. (n.d.). Physical activity for arthritis. CDC. https://www.cdc.gov/arthritis/basics/physical-activity/index.html

29. National Center for Biotechnology Information. (n.d.). Resistance exercise to prevent and manage sarcopenia and... https://www.ncbi.nlm.nih.gov/pmc/articles/PMC4849483/

30. Mayo Clinic. (n.d.). Exercise and chronic disease: Get the facts. Mayo Clinic. https://www.mayoclinic.org/healthy-lifestyle/fitness/in-depth/exercise-and-chronic-disease/art-20046049

31. Department of Physiology, University of Arizona, Tucson, AZ; & Exercise and Health Laboratory, Faculty of Human Movement, Technical University of Lisbon, Lisbon, PORTUGAL. (2002). Resistance Training in Postmenopausal Women with and without Hormone Therapy. Official Journal of the American College of Sports Medicine.

32. Grindler, Natalia M. MD; Santoro, Nanette F. MD. Menopause and exercise. Menopause 22(12):p 1351-1358, December 2015. | DOI: 10.1097/GME.0000000000000536

33. Mishra, Nalini; Mishra, V. N.1; Devanshi, 2. Exercise beyond menopause: Dos and Don'ts. Journal of Mid-life Health 2(2):p 51-56, Jul–Dec 2011. | DOI: 10.4103/0976-7800.92524

34. Layne JE, Arabelovic S, Wilson LB, et al. Community-Based Strength Training Improves Physical Function in Older Women With Arthritis. American Journal of Lifestyle Medicine. 2009;3(6):466-473. doi:10.1177/1559827609342061

35. Choudhry, D. N., Saleem, S., Hatim, S., & Irfan, R. (2024). The effect of resistance training in reducing hot flushes in post-menopausal women: A meta-analysis. *Journal of Bodywork and Movement Therapies, 39*, 335-342. https://doi.org/10.1016/j.jbmt.2025.03.018

36. Delaney, M. F. (2006). Strategies for the prevention and treatment of osteoporosis during early postmenopause. American Journal of Obstetrics and Gynecology, 194(2, Supplement), S12-S23.

37. Zehnacker, Carol Hamilton PT, DPT, MS1; Bemis-Dougherty, Anita PT, DPT, MAS2. Effect of Weighted Exercises on Bone Mineral Density in Post Menopausal Women A Systematic Review. Journal of Geriatric Physical Therapy 30(2):p 79-88, August 2007.

38. Wardell, A. (2024, May 14). The paradox of women's aging: Is it possible to feel more and less confident at the same time? Compassionate Feminism. Reviewed by T. Woods.

39. Is Reformer Pilates worth the hype? | PilatesByPamela. https://pilatesbypamela.com/blog/is-reformer-pilates-worth-the-hype/

40. Leyva, J. (2024, February 20). How do muscles grow? The science of muscle growth. Transformations. https://www.builtlean.com/muscles-grow/

41. Common Menopause Myths: Separating fact from fiction. (n.d.). https://www.nutritionnews.abbott/healthy-living/aging-well/Common-Menopause-Myths-Separating-Fact-From-Fiction/

42. Calorie calculator. (2022, November 29). Mayo Clinic. https://www.mayoclinic.org/healthy-lifestyle/weight-loss/in-depth/calorie-calculator/itt-20402304

43. Groves, M. (2023, December 4). Menopause Diet: How what you eat affects your symptoms. Healthline. https://www.healthline.com/nutrition/menopause-diet#foods-to-avoid

44. Blogs & news. (n.d.). Doctors at Kaiser Permanente in MD, VA, DC. https://mydoctor.kaiserpermanente.org/mas/news/menopause-diet-how-to-eat-right-to-avoid-weight-gain-2214485

45. UCLA Health. (2024, April 11). The best way to work out after menopause. https://www.uclahealth.org/news/article/best-way-work-out-after-menopause

46. Melmed, S., Polonsky, K. S., Larsen, P. R., & Kronenberg, H. M. (2016). *Williams Textbook of Endocrinology* (13th ed.). Elsevier.

47. Jameson, J. L., Fauci, A. S., Kasper, D. L., Hauser, S. L., Longo, D. L., & Loscalzo, J. (2018). *Harrison's Principles of Internal Medicine* (20th ed.). McGraw-Hill Education.

48. The North American Menopause Society. (2017). *The 2017 hormone therapy position statement of The North American Menopause Society*. Menopause, 24(7), 728-753. https://doi.org/10.1097/GME.0000000000000921

49. The Endocrine Society. (2015). *Management of menopause symptoms: Clinical practice guidelines*. The Journal of Clinical Endocrinology & Metabolism, 100(11), 3975-4011. https://doi.org/10.1210/jc.2015-2236

50. Santoro, N., & Randolph, J. F. (2011). Reproductive hormones and the menopause transition. *Journal of Clinical Endocrinology & Metabolism*, 96(11), 3648-3657. https://doi.org/10.1210/jc.2011-1047

51. Shifren, J. L., & Gass, M. L. S. (2014). The North American Menopause Society recommendations for clinical care of midlife women. *Menopause*, 21(10), 1038-1062. https://doi.org/10.1097/GME.0000000000000319

52. Mayo Clinic. (2021). *Menopause*. Mayo Clinic. https://www.mayoclinic.org/diseases-conditions/menopause/symptoms-causes/syc-20353397

53. The North American Menopause Society. (2017). *Hormone therapy position statement of The North American Menopause Society*. Menopause, 24(7), 728-753. https://doi.org/10.1097/GME.0000000000000921

54. Endocrine Society. (n.d.). Menopause. Retrieved July 23, 2024, from https://www.endocrine.org/patient-engagement/endocrine-library/menopause#:~:text=As%20women%20approach%20mid%2Dlife,to%20skip%20oher%20periods%20altogether.

55. American College of Sports Medicine. (2019). ACSM's guidelines for strength training. ACSM

56. National Institute on Aging. (n.d.). How can strength training build healthier bodies as we age? NIA

57. National Institute on Aging. (n.d.). Exercise and older adults toolkit. NIA

Made in the USA
Las Vegas, NV
27 December 2024

15458794R00074